A Choice Manual

A Choice Manual:
OR,
RARE and SELECT
SECRETS
IN
PHYSICK
AND
CHIRURGERY.

Collected and Practised by the Right Honourable the
Countess of KENT,
Lately DECEASED.

Whereto are added,
Several Experiments of the Virtues of *Gascon-Powder*, and *Lapis Contra Yarvam*; by a Professor of *Physick*.

As also most exquisite Ways of *Preserving, Conserving, Candying*, &c.

The 22d Edition, with ADDITIONS.

LONDON:
Printed for JOHN CLARKE, at the Golden Ball in Duck-Lane, 1726.

To the Virtuous and most Noble Lady, *Latitia Popham*, Wife of the Honourable, and truly Valiant Collonel *Alexander Popham*.

Thrice Noble and truly Vertuous Lady,

AFter mature deliberation, what to render unto your acceptance worthy your Patronage, nothing occurred more probable than this small Manual; which was once esteemed a rich Cabinet of knowledge, by a Person truly Honourable. May it auspitiously procure but your Honours like friendly estimation, and then I doubt not, but it will find a universal acceptance amongst Persons of greatest Eminency. Sure I am, it may be justly deemed as a rich Magazine of Experience, having long since taught the World it's approved excellency, yea, even in many dangerous exigencies.

A 2   All

The Epistle Dedicatory.

All I humbly crave for the present is, my boldness may be favourably excused, since 'twas my lawful ambition, thereby to avoid ingratitude, for the many singular favours I have already received from your endeared truly Honourable Husband, my always true noble Friend, and most happy Country-man. God multiply his Blessings upon all your noble Family, and make you no less honourable here on Earth, than eternally happy hereafter; which shall be the daily Prayer of him, whose highest E-mulation is,

In all due ways

abundantly to Honour

and Serve you,

W. J.

TO

TO THE READER.

Courteous Reader,

WEll remembring that we are all born for the Weal publick good: I here tender to thy perufal this fmall, and yet moſt excellent Treatife, Entituled, *A Choice Manual of Rare and Select Secrets in Phyſick*: If thereby you fuck abundance of profit, I ſhall be fuperlatively glad; but if any, or perchance many unlooked for miſtakes, for want of a due application bid thee entertain contrary thoughts, the effect not anſwering thy curious expectation, upon a more ferious reflex, know, that nothing is abfolutely perfect, and withal, that the richeſt and moſt foveraign Antidote may be often mifapplied: wherefore the fault not being mine, excufe and ceaſe to cenfure: For which juſt and but reaſonable favour, thou ſhalt defervedly oblige me,

Thine W. J.

A Table of the Contents.

A

For an Ague   13,32,67,71,76
For an Ach   14,19,29,30,51,59,63,72,80
Aqua Composita   56,62,67
For an Ach in the Back   63
For a Tertian Ague   76
For the stinging of an Adder   ibid.
Mr Ashley's Ointment   79
For an Ach in the Joint   62
The Virtue of Aqua Bezoar   93
Spirit of Confection of Alkermes with its Virtues   96
Extract of Ambergriece   ibid.

B

For a Bruise   5,15,28,37,38,46,48,51,54,73
A restoring Broth   10
A strengthening Meat for the same   ibid.
A Cordial for a Breakfast   11
For a griping of the Belly   ibid
To clear the Blood   16
For burning in the Back   ibid.
For weakness in the Back   17,50
For a sore Breast   19
For a stinking Breath   16,19
For one that pisseth Blood   24
For the Bone-ach   14,31,72
For a burning by Lightning   41
To stench Blood   42
For the Black Jaundice   43

For

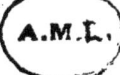

The Contents

For Burning with Gun-powder	41,47
A plaister for the Back	38,39,56
To make Balm-water	54 70
For an inward Bruising	28,73
For a Blast	82
Balsamum	ibid.

C

For a Consumption and Cough of the Lungs	1,14,48,65
Cordials	8,38
To make a Jelly and Glister for the Cough	7
For an extream Cough and Cold	6,87
China Broth for a Consumption	12
Another Broth for a Consumption	10,13
For Corns	25
For a Canker	26,51,58,74
For pain after Child-birth	33
For swollen Cods	34
For the Cholick	50,67
For all manner of Cuts	35,49
For a dead Child in a Woman	45,76
To deliver a Child in danger	65
To cool Choller	66
For the Cholick-passion	67
For Children that are troubled with an extream Cough	73,87
For a Cold	17,82
Powder of Crabs-claws	90
The Virtues of a Root call'd Contra Yarva	91
Virtues of Spirit of Clary	94
Virtues of Spirit of Comfrey	96

D

For the Dropsie	16
For the biting of a mad Dog	31,36,76
Virtue of Spirit of Diasatyrion	95

E

For all Infirmities and Diseases of the Eyes	15, 18 24 25,53 72,73,84 85
For a Pin, and Web, and redness in the Eye	37,72

For

The Contents

For the Emerhoids	47,63,74
For the Rheum at the Eyes	62
For fore Eyes	16,53,64
Several Experiments made of the Countess of Kents Powder	97

F

For Faintness	2
For Flegm	6
To know whether he that hath the Flux shall live or die	23
For the Falling sickness	2,27,83
For the Bloody-flux	28,67,84
To kill a Fellon	32,57,60,63
To break a Fellon	57,63
Oyl of Foxes its Virtues	51
Jelly of Frogs	86
For a red Face	88

G

For the Gout	21,45
For the Green-Sickness	41
Gascons Powder	89
Gascons Powder for the Apothecaries	90
To make a Glister	8

H

To make Horse-Radish Drink	4
To take away Hoarsness	7
To take away Head-ach	ibid.
A Cordial for the Heart	42,43
For coldness in the Head	17
For Hearing	22,44,60
For the breaking out of Childrens Heads	27
For the swelling of the Head with a Fall	34
For a new Hurt	35
To cleanse the Head	36
For singing in the Head	48
For a Heat, burning or scalding	61
Oyl of Hypericon	83
For a scald Head	60,84

For

The Contents

For Heat of the foles of the Feet	61,89

I

For the Itch	6,46,84
Oyl of St. John' Wort	39
For a ftrain in the Joints	71,78,80
Jelly of Hart's-horn	7

K

For Kibes	13,83
The Countefs of Kent's Powder	91

L

For the Liver	6,42,56
For a Lask	34 46,55,58
To caufe eafie Labour	38
Againft grief of the Lungs	43,49,65
To keep ones body loofe	88

M

Againft Melancholy	2,4,35,55
Aqua Mirabilis, with the Virtues	3
To prevent Mifcarrying	13
For the Mother	53 74
The Virtues of Aqua Mariæ	94
The Virtues of Spirit of Mints	ibid.
The Compofitum of Oleum Magiftrale	100

P

For the Plague	5,48,52,53,68,75,86,87
For the Plurifie	13 36
For a dead Palfie	19,50
A good Purge	20,29,43
For a prick with a Nail or Thorn	47,52,57
To make the leaden Plaifter	51
The Virtue of the Plaifter	52
For the Ptifik	59
For pricking and burning in the foles of the Feet	61
For a pufh	63
The beft Paracelfus Salve	77
A Excellent Plague-water	81
A defenfive Plaifter againft the Plague	81

R

Running

The Contents

Running of the Reins	17,34,40,61.82
Pectoral Rolls	17
For the Reins of the Back	30,51
For all sorts of Rheums	46.62
For one that hath a Rupture	48,49,57
Virtues of Flowers of Rosemary	94
Virtues of Spirits of Roses	95

S

For Stone in the Kidnies	2,4,37,43,55
A Medicine for those that are sick after eating	66
For a Stitch	30, 48
For Scabs	6
For the Scurvy	16
To strengthen the Stomack	20,42,64
For Sun-burnt	17
For a Swelling or Sore	19 25,26,56
For spitting of Blood	23,35,36,49
Against surfeiting	24,30,54,85
For Sinews that are shrunk	31,67
Dr. Stephens's Water	32,70
To cause one to sleep	50,58,60
For pain in the Stomack	37,59
A Cordial for the Sea	28
For the Stone	46,55,66
For an old Sore, or other Sores	39,42,44,46,49,58, 61,63 80
To make Oyl of sage	42
For a Scald	47,61,74
To make Oyl of Swallows	57
For the Sight	18,59
For the stiffness of the Sinews	67
For the spleen	42,73
Virtues of Spirit of Saffron	95
Virtues of Spirit of Strawberries	ibid.

T

For stopping in the Throat	6
To distill Treacle water	ibid.
For a Tetter	28,47,88

To

The Contents

To keep Teeth clean	42
To cure the Garget in the Throat	44
To quench Thirst	59
For the Tooth-ach	43.86
To fasten the Teeth	87
To make one taste their Meat	ibid.
The Virtues of Aqua Theriacilis	94

V

How to stay Vomiting	17
How to stop the bleeding of a Vein	23,36
For a Vein ill smitten	24
For Ulcers	27
Flos Unguentorum	28
Against biting of Venemous Beasts	34
Against falling of the Uvula	89

W

A Cordial for the Wind in the stomach	8 50,71
Restoratives for the same	9
For a green Wound or other Wounds	31,34,35,40 53,61,65
For one that is Weak	55
To stench bleeding of a Wound	82
For a Woman travelling with Child	39
For a Wen	27
For cankered Wounds	31
Dr. Willoughbee's Water	33
To draw an Arrow-head, or any Iron out of a Wound	34
For a Woman that hath her Flowers too much	45
To cause a Woman to have her sickness	46
To kill Worms	46,75
For the Wind-Chollick	50,76
For one that cannot make Water	56,89
To take away Warts	59

Y

Yellow Jaundice	18

A CHOICE MANUAL,
OR,
RARE and SELECT
SECRETS
IN
PHYSICK.

A very good Medicine for a Consumption, and Cough of the Lungs.

TAke a Pound of the best Honey you can get, and dissolve it in a Pipkin, then take it off the fire, and put in two pennyworth of flower of Brimstone, and two pennyworth of powder of *Elecampana*, and two pennyworth of the flower of Liquorice, and two pennyworth of red Rose-water, and so stir them together, till they be all compounded together, and put it into a gallypot, and when you use it, take a Liquorice stick beaten at one end, and take up with it as much almost as half a Walnut, at night when you go to bed, and in the morning fasting, or at any time in the night when you are troubled with the Cough, and so let it melt down in your mouth by degrees.

Sir John Digbies Medicine for the Stone in the Kidneys.

Take a pound of the finest Honey, and take seven quarts of Conduit-water, set them on the fire, and when it is ready to seeth, scum it, and still as the froth doth rise, scum it, and put in 20 whole Cloves, and let them seeth softly for the space of half an hour, and so bottle it up for your use, and drink it morning and evening, and at your meat, and use no other drink until you are well.

A Medicine for the Falling-sickness.

Take a penny weight of the powder of Gold, six penny weight of Pearl, six penny weight of Amber, six penny weight of Corral, eight grains of Bezar, half an ounce of Piony seeds; also you must put some powder of a dead mans skull, that hath been an Anatomy, for a Woman, and the powder of a Woman for a Man, compound all these together; and take as much of the powder of all these as will lie upon a two-pence for nine mornings together in Endive-water, and drink a good draught of Endive water after it.

For Cordials and Restoratives use these things following.

In any faintness, take three drops of Oil of Cinnamon, mixed with a spoonful of syrup of Gilliflowers, and as much Cinnamon-water; drink this for a Cordial.

Against Melancholy.

Take one spoonful of Gilliflowers, the weight of seven Barly-corns of Bever-stone, bruise it as fine as flower, and so put it into two spoonfuls of syrup of Gilliflowers, and take it four hours after Supper, or else four hours after Dinner, this will chear the heart.

If you be sick after meat, use this.

Take of the best green Ginger that is preserved in syrup, shred it in small pieces, put it into a gallypot, and put Cinnamon water to it, then after dinner or supper eat the quantity of two Nutmegs upon a Knifes point.

Aqua Mirabilis.

Take three pints of White wine, one pint of *Aqua vitæ*, one pint of juice of Celendine, one dram of Cardamar, a dram of Melilot-flowers, Cubebs a dram, of Galingal, Nutmeg, Mace, Ginger, and Cloves, of each a dram; mingle all these together over night, the next morning set them a stilling in a glass Limbeck.

The Virtues.

This Water dissolveth swelling of the Lungs, and being perished doth help and comfort them, it suffereth not the blood to putrifie, he shall not need to be let blood that useth this water, it suffereth not the heart-burning, nor Melancholy or Flegm to have dominion, it expelleth Urine, and profiteth the stomach, it preserveth a good colour, the visage, memory, and youth, it destroyeth the Palsie.

Take some three spoonfuls of it once or twice a Week, or oftner, morning and evening, first and last.

Another way to make Aqua Mirabilis.

Take Galingal, Cloves, Quibs, Ginger, Mellilip, Cardamony, Mace, Nutmegs, of each a dram, and of the juice of Celendine half a pint, adding the juice of Mints and Balm, of each half a pint more, and mingle all the said Spices, being beaten into a powder with the juice, with a pint of good *Aqua vitæ*, and three pints of good White-wine, and put all these together into a pot, and let it stand all night being close stopt, and in the morn-ing,

ing still it with a soft fire as can be, the still being close pasted, and a cold still.

A Medicine for the Stone in the Kidneys.

Take a good handful of Pellitory of the wall, a handful of Mead, Parsley, Saxifrage, a handful of wild Thyme, a handful of Garden Parsley, three spoonfuls of Fennel-seeds, six Horse Raddish Roots sliced, then shred all these together, put them in a gallon of new Milk, and let them stand and steep in a close pot one whole night, and then still them, Milk and all together, this must be done in *May* or *June*, for then Hearbs are in their best State; and when it is taken you must put two or three spoonfuls of this water, as much white Wine as Renish, and if you please a little Sugar, and so take it two days before the Change, and two days after, and two days before the Full, and two days after, continuing taking the same all the Year, and the Patient undoubtedly shall find great Ease, and void many Stones, and much gravel, with little pain.

To make Horse-Raddish drink.

Take half a pound of Horse-Raddish, then wash and scrape them very clean, and slice them very thin cross ways on the Root, then put them into six quarts of small Ale, such as is ready for drinking, which being put into a pipkin close covered, set on the Embers, keeping it little more than blood warm for twelve hours, then take it off the fire, and let it stand to cool until the next morning, then pour the clear Liquor into bottles, and keep it for your use, drinking a good draught thereof in the Morning, fasting two hours after, and the like quantity at Four in the Afternoon, this drink is excellent good against Winds, as also for the Scouring and Dropsie, being taken in time.

An excellent Sirrup against Melancholy.

Take four quarts of the juice of Pearmains, and twice as much of the juice of Buglofs and Borrage, if they be to be gotten, a drachm of the best English Saffron, bruise it, and put it into the juice, then take two drachms of *Kermes* small beaten to pouder, mix it also with the juice, so being mixt, put them into an earthen vessel, covered or stopt forty eight hours, then strain it, and allow a pound of Sugar to every quart of juice, and so boil it to the Ordinary height of a Sirrup, after it is boiled, take one drachm of the spices of Diamber, and two drachms of the spices of *Diamargariton frigidum*, and so sew the same slenderly in a Linnen bag, that you may put the same easily into the bottle of sirrup, and so let it hang with a thread out at the mouth of the bottle; the spices must be put into the sirrup in the bag, so soon as the sirrup is off the fire, whilst it is hot, then afterwards put it into the bottle, and there let it hang: put but a spoonful or two of Honey amongst it while it is boiling, and it will make the scum rise, and the sirrup very clear.

You must add to it the quantity of a quarter of a pint of the Juyce of Balm.

An excellent Receit for the Plague.

Take one pound of green Walnuts, half an ounce of Saffron, and half an ounce of *London* Triacle, beaten together in a Mortar, and with a little *Carduus*, or some such water, vapour it over the fire, till it come to an Electuary: keep this in a pot, and take as much as a Walnut; it is good to cure a Feaver, Plague, and any Infection.

An excellent Cordial.

Take the flowers of Marigolds, and lay them in small spirit of Wine, when the tincture is fully taken out, pour it off from the flowers, and vapour it away till it come to a Consistence as thick as an Electuary.

For a bruise or stitch under the Ribs.

Take five or six handfuls of Cabbage, stamp it and strain it, after it is boiled in a quart of fair water, then sweeten it with Sugar, and drink it oft in a Wine glass in the morning, and at 4 in the afternoon, for five or six days together, then take a Cabbage-leaf, and between two dishes stew it, being wet first in Canary Wine, and that lay hot to your side evening and morning

An excellent Receit for an Itch, or any foul Scabs.

Take fox Gloves, and boil a handful of them in posset drink, and drink of it a draught at night, and in the Morning, then boil a good quantity of the Fox-gloves in fair running water, and anoint the places that are sore with the Water.

A Receit good for the Liver.

Take Turpentine, slice it thin, and lay it on a Silver or Purslane Plate, twice or thrice in the Oven with the Bread, till it be dry, and so make it into pouder, every day take as much as will lye on a six-pence in an Egg.

For Flegm, and stopping in the Throat and Stomach. D.T.

Take Oil of Almonds, Linseed Oil, buds of Orange flowers, boil all these in Milk, and anoint the stomach well with it, and lay a scarlet cloth next to it.

For an extream Cold, and a Cough.

Take of Hysop water six ounces, of red Poppy-water four ounces, six Dates, ten Figs, and slice them small, a handful of Raisins of the Sun, the weight of a Shilling of the powder of Liquorice; put these into the aforesaid waters, and let them stand five or six hours upon warm embers close covered, and not boil, then strain forth the water, and put into it as much Sugar of Roses as will sweeten it : drink of this in the morning, and at four of the clock in the afternoon, and when you go to bed.

To distill Triacle-water.

Take one ounce of Harts-horn shaved, and boil it in three pints of *Carduus* water till it come to a quart, then take the Roots Elecampane, Centian,

Ciprefs, Turmentil, and of Citron rinds, of each one ounce, Borrage, Buglofs, Rofemary flowers, of each two ounces; then take a pound of the beft old Triacle, and diffolve it in 6 pints of White-wine, and three pints of Rofe-water, fo infufe all together, and diftil it.

It is good to reftore Spirits, and fpeech, and good againft fwouning, Faintnefs, Agues, and Worms, and the fmall Pox.

Triacle-water.

Take three ounces of *Venice* Triacle, and mingle it in a quart of fpirits of wine, fet it in horfe-dung four or five days, then ftill it in afhes, or fand twice over; after take the bottom which is left in the Still, and put to it a pint of fpirit of Wine, and fet it in the dung till the tincture be clean out of it, and fet it on the fire, till it become to be a thick confiftence, it muft be kept with a foft fire. And fo the like with Saffron.

To take away Hoarfnefs.

Take a Turnip, cut a hole in the top of it, and fill it up with brown Sugar-candy, and fo roaft it in the embers, and eat it with butter.

To take away the Head-ach.

Take the beft Sallade Oil, and the glafs half full with tops of Poppy-flowers which groweth in the Corn; fet this in the Sun a Fortnight, and fo keep it all the year, and anoint the Temples of your head with it.

For a Cough.

Take Sallade Oil, *Aqua vitæ*, and Sack, of each an equal quantity, beat them all together, and before the fire rub the foles of your feet with it.

To make Jelley of Harts-horn.

Take a quart of running water, and three ounces of Harts-horn fcraped very fine, then put it into a ftone Jug, and fet the Jug in a Kettle of water over the fire, and let it boil two or three hours until

until it Jelly, then put it into 3 or 4 spoonfuls of Rosewater, or White-wine, then strain it: you may put into it Musk, or Ambergreece, and season it as you please.

To make a Glister.

Take half a quart of new Milk, or three quarters, set it on the fire, and make it scalding hot, then take it off, and put into it the yolk of a new laid Egg beaten, two ounces of brown Sugar-candy, or black Sugar, give it to the party blood-warm.

Another.

Take the bone of a neck of Mutton, or Veal, clean washed, set it on the fire to boil in three pints of fair water, and when it is clean scummed, then put in the Roots of Fennel and Parsley clean washed and scraped, of either of them, the Roots bruised a handful, of Cammomil and Mallows a handful, let all these boil together till half be wasted, then strain it; take three quarters of a pint of this broth, brown Sugar-candy two ounces, of Oil of Flax-seed two ounces; mingle all these together, and take it for a Glister blood-warm, when it is in your body, keep it half an hour, or three quarters of an hour, or an hour if you can.

A comfortable Cordial to chear the Heart.

Take one ounce of Conserve of Cilliflowers, 4 grains of the best Musk bruised as fine as flower; then put it into a little tin pot, and keep it till you have need to make this Cordial following; viz. Take the quantity of one Nutmeg out of your tin pot, put to it one spoonful of Cinnamon water, and one spoonful of the sirrup of Gilliflowers, Ambergriece; mix all these together, and drink them in the morning, Fasting 3 or 4 hours: this is most comfortable.

A Cordial for Wind in the stomach, or any part.

Take six or eight spoonfuls of Penniroyal-water, put into it four drops, of Oil of Cinnamon, so drink it any time of the day, so you fast two hours after.

Restoratives.

Take a well flesht Capon from the Barn door, and pluck out his Intrals, then wash it within with a little white-Wine, then fley off all the skin, and take out his bones, and take the flesh, only cut it in little pieces, and put it into a little stone bottle, and put to it one ounce of white Sugar-candy, six Dates slit, with the stones and piths taken out, one large Mace, then stop the bottle up fast, and set it in a Chafer of water, and let it boil three hours; then take it out, and pour the juice from the meat, and put to it one spoonful of red rose-water, and take the better part for your breakfast 4 hours before dinner, and the other part at three a clock in the afternoon, being blood-warm.

Another Restorative.

Take half a pint of Claret wine, and half a pint of Ale, and make a Caudle with a new laid Egg; put in half a nutmeg cut in two pieces, then take it off the fire, and put in seven grains of Ambergriece; drink this for two Breakfasts, for it will encrease blood and strength.

Another Restorative.

Take two new-laid Eggs, and take the whites clean from them, and put the yolks both in one shell; then put in two spoonfuls of Claret wine, seven grains of Ambergriece small bruised, and a little Sugar-Candy; stir all these together, and make them blood-warm, and sup them up for a breakfast three or four hours before Dinner.

Another Restorative.

Take a young leg of Mutton, cut off the skin and the Fat, take the flesh being cut into small pieces, and put it into a stone bottle, then put to it two ounces of Raisins of the Sun stoned, a large Mace, an ounce an half of Sugar-candy, and stop the bottle close,

close, and let it boil in a Chafer three hours, and so put the juice from the meat, and keep it in a clean glass; it will serve for three breakfasts, or if he will he may take some at three of the clock in the Afternoon being made warm.

A Restoring Broth.

Take 2 ounces of Chene-roots, first slit very thin, then put it in a new Pipkin with five pints of running water being close covered, and so set it upon Embers all night long, where it may be very hot, but not seeth; then put to that water a great Cock Chicken, and when it is clean scummed, put into it two spoonfuls of French Barly, six Dates slit, with the piths and stones taken out, two ounces of Raisins of the Sun ston'd, a large Mace, let all these boil together till half be consumed, then take out the *Cock,* and beat the flesh of it in a clean Mortar and a little of the broth, then strain it altogether throughout a hair Cullender, then put in two spoonfuls of red Rose-water, and sweeten it with white Sugar-candy; drink of this Broth, being made warm, half a pint in the morning early fasting, and sleep after it if you can, drink a good draught at three of the clock in the afternoon; this broth is very good for a Consumption, and the longer they take it, it is the better.

A strengthening Meat.

Take Potato-roots, roast them or bake them, then pill them, and slice them into a dish, put to it lumps of raw Marrow, and a few Currans, a little whole Mace, and sweeten it with Sugar to your taste, and and so eat it instead of buttered Parsnips.

Broth for a Consumption.

Take three Marrow bones, break them in pieces, and boil them in a Gallon of water till half be consumed, then strain the liquor through a Cullender, and let it stand while it be cold, then take off all the Fat clean, and put the broth into a pipkin, and put

put to it a good Cock chicken, and a Knuckle of Veal, then put into it the bottom of a white loaf, a whole Mace, two ounces of Raisins of the Sun stoned, six Dates slit; let all these boil together till half be consumed, then strain it; instead of Almonds take a few Pistaties kernels and beat them, and strain with your Broths as you do Almond-milk, and so sweeten it with white sugar, and drink half a pint early in the Morning and at three a Clock in the Afternoon, and so continue a good while together, or else it would do you no good.

Another Cordial.

Take a preserved Nutmeg, cut it in four quarters, eat a quarter at a Breakfast, and another in the Afternoon; this is good for the Head and Stomach.

A Cordial for a Breakfast fasting.

Eat a good piece of a Pomecition preserved, as big as your two fingers in length and breadth, and so at three of the Clock in the Afternoon.

A Restoring Breakfast.

Take the Brawn of a Capon, or Pullet, twelve Jordan Almonds blanched, beat them together, and strain out the juice with a draught of strong Broth, and take it for a Breakfast, or to bedward.

A Medicine for any griping of the Belly.

Take a pint of Claret-wine, put to it a spoonful of Parsley-seed, and a spoonful of sweet Fennel-seed, half a dozen Cloves, a branch of Rosemary, a wild Mallow-root clean washt and scrapt, and the pith taken out, with a good piece of sugar; set this on the fire, and burn the Claret very well with all these things in it, then drink a good draught of it in the morning Fasting, and at three a clock in the Afternoon.

To keep the Body Laxative.

Take half a pint of running Water, put it in a new Pipkin with a cover, then put into the Water two ounces of Manna, and when it is dissolved, strain

strain it, and put to it four ounces of Damask Prunes, eight Cloves, a branch of Rosemary; let all these stew together while they be very tender, then eat a dozen of them with a little of the Liquor an hour before Dinner or Supper, then take a draught of Broth and Dine.

To make the China *Broth for a Consumption.*

Take *China* root thin sliced two ounces, steep it 24 hours, in eight pints of fair water, letting it stand warm all the time, being close covered in an earthen Pipkin, or Iron pot; then put to it a good Cockrel, or two Chickens clean dressed, and scum it well, then put in five-leaved grass two handfuls, Maiden-hair, Harts tongue, of either half a handful, twenty Dates sliced, two or three Mace, and the bottom of a Manchet, let all these stew together, until not above one quart remains, then strain it, and take all the flesh, and sweet bones: beat them in a stone Mortar, and strain out all the juice with the Broth; then sweeten it with two ounces of white Sugar-candy in pouder, and take thereof half a pint at once, early in the morning warm, and sleep after it if you can, and two hours before Supper at your pleasure; when you steep the Root, slice two drachms of white Sanders, and as much red Sanders, and let them boil in the Broth.

A gentle Purge

Take an ounce of Damask Roses, eat it all at one time, fast three quarters of an hour after, then take a draught of Broth and dine.

Another Purge.

Take the weight of four or five pence, of Rubarb, cut it in little pieces, and take a spoonful or two of good Currans washt very clean, so mingle them together, and so eat them, fast an hour after, and begin that meal with broth, you may take it an hour before if you will.

Broth for a Consumption.

Take a courſe Pullet, and ſow up the belly, and an ounce of the Conſerves of Red Roſes, of the Conſerves of Borrage and Bugloſs flowers, of each of them half a ounce, Pine-Apple kernels, and Piſtaties, of each half an ounce bruiſed in a Mortar, two drachms of Amber powder, all mixed together, and put in the belly, then boil it in three quarts of Water with Egrimony, Endive, and Succory, of each one handful, Sparrow-graſs-roots, Fennel-roots, Caper-roots, and one handful of Raiſins of the Sun ſtoned; when it is almoſt boiled, take out the Pullet, and beat it in a ſtone Mortar; then put it into the liquor again, and give it 3 or 4 walms more, then ſtrain it, and put to it a little Red roſe water, and half a pint of White-wine, and ſo drink it in a morning, and ſleep after it.

To prevent miſcarrying.

Take Venice Turpentine, ſpread it on brown Paper, the bredth and length of a hand; lay it to the ſmall of her back, then give her to drink a Caudle made of Muskadine, and put into it the husks of 23 ſweet Almonds dryed, and finely poudered.

For Boiles, or Kibes, or to draw a Sore.

Take ſtrong Ale, and boil it from a pint to four ſpoonfuls, and ſo keep it, it will be an Ointment.

To make Cammomil Oil.

Shred a pound of Cammomil, and knead it into a pound of ſweet Butter, melt it, and ſtrain it.

A Receipt for the Pluriſie.

Take three round Balls of Horſe-dung; boil them in a pint of White-wine till half be conſumed, then ſtrain it out, and ſweeten it with a little Sugar, and let the patient go to bed, and drink this, then lay him warm.

For an Ague.

Take a pint of Milk, and ſet it on the fire, and when it boils put in a pint of Ale, then take off the

Curd and put in nine heads of *Carduus*, let it boil till half be wasted, then to every quarter of a pint, put a good spoonful of Wheat-flower, and a quarter of a spoonful of gross Pepper, and an hour before the Fit, let the Patient drink a quarter of a pint, and be sure to lye in a sweat before the Fit.

An excellent Balm for a green Wound.

Take two good handfuls of English Tobacco, shred it small, and put it into a pint of Sallade-oil, and seeth it on a soft fire to simper, till the Oil change green; then strain it, and in the cooling put in two ounces of *Venice* Turpentine.

For an Ach

Take of the best Gall, White-wine Vinegar, and *Aqua vitæ*, of each a like quantity, and boil it gently on the fire, till it grow clammy, then put it in a glass or pot, and when you use any of it, warm it against the fire, rub some of it with your hand on the aking place, and lay a linnen cloath on it; do this mornings and evenings.

To make a Searcloth.

Virgins Wax, *Sperma Ceti*, *Venice* Turpentine, Oil of white Poppy, Oil of Ben, Oil of sweet Almonds.

For Wind in the Stomach and the Spleen

Take a handful of Bloom, and boil it in a pint of beer or Ale till it be half consumed, and drink it for the Wind, and the Stomach, and for the Spleen.

A most excellent Water for a Consumption, and Cough of the Lungs.

Take a running Cock, pull him alive, then kill him, when he is almost cold cut him abroad by the back, and take out the Intrals, and wipe him clean, then cut him in quarters, and break the bones, put him into such a Still as you still use water in, and with a pottle of Sack, a pound of Currans, a pound of Raisins of the Sun, stoned, a quarter of
a

a pound of Dates, the stones taken out, and the Dates cut small, two handfuls of wild Thyme, two handfuls of Orgares, two handfuls of Pimperbal, and two handfuls of Rosemary, two handfuls of Buglosse and Borrage-flowers, a bottle of new Milk of a red Cow; still this with a soft fire, put into the glass that the water doth drop into, half a pound of Sugar-candy beaten very small, one Book of leaf gold cut small among the Sugar, four grains of Ambergriece, twelve grains of prepared Pearl, you must mingle the strong water with the small, and drink four spoonfuls at a time in the morning Fasting, and an hour before supper; you must shake about the glass when you drink it.

For a Bruise.

Take six spoonfuls of Honey, a great handful of Linseed, bruise these in a Mortar, and boil them in a pint of Milk an hour, then strain it very hard, and anoint your breast and stomach with it every morning and evening, and lay a red cloth upon it.

The Eye-water for the infirmities and Diseases of the Eye.

Take of the distilled water of the white wild Rose, half a pound of the distilled water of Celendine, Fennel, Eye-bright, and Rue, of each two ounces, of Cloves an ounce and a half, of white Sugar-candy one drachm, of *Tutia* prepared four ounces, pulverize all these Ingredients each by themselves, saving that you must bruise the Camphire with your Sugar-candy, for so it breaks best; then mix all the Pouders together in a paper, put them in a strong glass, pour the distilled waters upon them, and three pints of the best French White-wine that can be had, shake it every day three or four times long together for a month, and then you may use it: remember to keep it very close stopt. This is *verbatim* as it was had from the Lord *Kelly*.

A Medicine very good for the Dropsie, or the Scurvy, and to clear the Blood.

Take four gallons of ale drawn from the tap into an earthen Stand, when the Ale is two days old, then you must put in of Brook-lime, of Water-cresses, of water-mints with red stalks, of each four handfuls, half a peck of Scurvy-grass, let all these be clean picked, and washed, and dryed with a cloth, and shed with a Knife, and then put into a bag, then put in the Ale and stop it close, so that it have no vent, stop it with Rie paste; the best Scurvy grass groweth by the water side, it must be seven days after the things be in before you drink it. Take two quarts of water, and in four ounces of *Guiacum*, two ounces of Sarsaparilla, one ounce of Saxifrage, put it into a pipkin, and infuse it upon the embers for twelve hours, and then strain it, and put it into the Ale as soon as it hath done working, this being added makes the more Caudle.

For sore Eyes.

Take half a pint of red rose water, put therein four penny-worth of Aloe succatrina, as much *Bole armoniac* in quantity, let this lye four and twenty hours in steep, then wash your eye with it evenings and mornings with a Feather, and it will help them.

A Sirrup to strengthen the Stomach, and the Brain, and to make a sweet Breath.

Take Rinds while they be new one pound, of running water the value of five Wine pints, then seeth it unto 3 pints, then strain it, and with one pound of Sugar, seeth it to a Sirrup, and when you take it from the fire, put to it 4 grains of Musk.

For the burning in the Back.

Take the juice of Plantain, and Womans Milk, being of a Woman Child, put thereto a spoonful of Rose-water, and wet a fine cloth in the same, and so lay it to your back where the heat is.

Rare Secrets in Physick.

A very good Medicine to stay the Vomiting.

Take of Spear-mints, Worm-wood, and red Rose-leaves dryed, of each half a handful, of Rye-bread grated a good handful, boil all these in red Rose-water and Vinegar, till they be somewhat tender, then put it into a linnen cloth, and lay it to the stomach as hot as you can endure it, heating it two or three times a Day with such as it was boiled in.

For weakness in the Back.

Take Nip, and Clary, and the Marrow of an Ox-back, chop them very small, then take the yolks of two or three Eggs, and strain them all together, then fry them; use this six or seven times together, and after it drink a good draught of Bastard or Muskadine.

To make a Cap for the Pain and Coldness of the Head.

Take of Storix and Benjamine, of both some twelve penniworth, and bruise it, then quilt it in a brown Paper, and wear it behind on your Head.

To make pectoral Rouls for a Cold.

Take four Ounces of Sugar finely beaten, and half an Ounce of searched Liquorice, two Grains of Musk, and the weight of two Pence of the Sirrup of Liquorice, and so beat it up to a perfect Paste, with a little Sirrup of Horehound, and a little Guindragon being steeped in Rose water, then roul them in small Rouls and dry them, and so you may keep them all the year.

For the running of the Reins.

Take the pith of an Ox that goeth down the back, a pint of red Wine, and strain them together through a cloth, then boil them a little with a good quantity of Cinnamon, and a Nutmeg, and a large Mace, a quantity of Ambergriece; drink this first and last daily.

For Sun-burn.

Take the juice of a Lemon, and a little Bay Salt,

Salt, and wash your hands with it, and let them dry of themselves, wash them again, and you shall find all the spots and stains gone.

For a Pin, and Web, and redness in the Eye.

Take a pint of white Rose-water, half a pint of white Wine, as much of *Lapis Calaminaris* as a Walnut bruised, put all these in a glass, and set them in the Sun one week, and shake the Glass every day; then take it out of the Sun, and use it as you shall need.

A special Medicine to preserve the Sight.

Take of brown Fennel, Honeysuckles of the hedg, of wild Dasie roots picked, and washed, and dried, of Pearl-wort, of Eyebright, of red Roses, the white clipped away, of each of these a handful dry gathered, then steep all these herbs in a quart or Three Pints of the best White-wine in an earthen pot, and so let it lye in steep two or three daies close covered, stirring it three times a day, and so still it with a gentle fire, making two distillings, and so keep it for your use.

A proved Medicine for the Yellow Jaundice.

Take a pint of Muskadine, a pretty quantity of the inner bark of a Barberry-tree, three spoonfuls of the greenest Goose-dung, you can get, and take away all the white Spots of it, lay them in steep all Night, on the Morrow strain it, and put to it one grated Nutmeg, one penniworth of Saffron dryed, and very finely beaten, and give it to Drink in the Morning

To make Pectoral Rouls.

Take one Pound of fine Sugar, of Liquorice, and Anise-seeds two spoonfuls, Elecampane one spoonful, of Amber, and Corral, of each a quarter of a spoonful, all this must be very finely beaten and searced, and then the quantity that is set down must be taken; mix all these powders together well, then take the white of an Egg, and beat it with a pretty quantity of Musk; then take a brazen Mortar very well scoured, and a spoonful or two of the Powders, and drop some of the Egg to it, so beat them to a paste, then make them in little rouls, and lay them on a place to dry.

A Plaister for a sore Breast.

Take crums of White-bread, the tops of Mint chopped small, and boil them in strong Ale, and make it like a Poultess, and when it is almost boiled, put in the Powder of Ginger, and Oil of Thyme, so spread it upon a Cloth, it will both Draw and Heal.

A Medicine for the Dead Palsie, and for them that have lost their Speech.

Take Borrage-leaves, Marigold-leaves, or Flowers, of each a good Handful, boil it in a good Ale Posset, the Patient must drink a good draught of it in the Morning, and Sweat; if it be in the Arms or Leggs, they must be chafed for an Hour or two when they be grieved, and at Meals they must drink of no other drink till their Speech come to them again, and in Winter, if the Herbs be not to be had, the Seeds will serve.

An approved Medicine for an Ach, or Swelling.

Take the Flowers of Cammomil, and Rose-leaves, of each of them a like quantity, and seeth them in White-wine, and make a Plaister thereof, and let it be laid as Hot as may be suffered to the place grieved, and this will ease a Pain, and asswage the Swelling.

An approved Medicine for a Stinking Breath.

Take a good quantity of Rosemary-leaves and Flowers, and boil them in White-wine, and with a little Cinnamon and Benjamin beaten in Powder being put thereto, let the Patient use to wash his Mouth very often therewith, and this will presently help him.

A Choice Manual, or,

A good Broth for one that is Weak.

Take part of a Neck of Lamb, and a pretty running Fowl, and set them on the Fire in fair Spring Water, and when it boileth Scum it well, so done, put in two large Mace, and a few Raisins of the Sun stored, and a little Fennel-root, and a Parsley-root, and let them boil; if the Party be grieved with heat or cold in the Stomach, if Heat, put in a Handful of Barley boiled before in two Waters, and some Violet-leaves, Sorrel, Succory, and a little Egrimony; if Cold, put in Rosemary, Thyme, a Lilly, Marigold-leaves, Borrage, and Bugloss, and boil this from four pints to less than one.

A Receit for Purging D. T.

Take the Leaves of new Sene six Ounces, of chosen Rubarb one Ounce and Half, Leaves of Sage, and Dock roots, of each an Ounce, of Barberries half an Ounce, Cinnamon, and Nutmeg, of each an Ounce, Annise-seeds, and Fennel-seeds, of each six Drams, of Tamarisk half an Ounce, Cloves and Mace, of each half a Dram, beat them into a gross Powder, and hang them in a Linnen Bag in six Gallons of new Ale, so Drink it Fasting in the Morning, and at Night.

To Comfort the Stomach, and help Windiness and Rheum.

Take of Ginger one Penniworth, Cloves four Penniworth, Mace seven Penniworth, Nutmeg four Penny-worth, Cinnamon four Penny-worth, and Galingal two Penny-worth, of each an Ounce, of Cubebs, Corral, and Amber, of each two Drams, of Fennel-seeds, Dill-seed, and Caraway-seed, of each one Ounce, of Liquorice and Annise-seeds, of each one Ounce, all beaten into fine Powder, one Pound and a Half of Fine beaten Sugar, which must be set on a soft Fire, and being dissolved, the Powders being well mixed therewith till it be stiff, then put thereunto Half a Pint of red Rose-water, and mix them well together, and put

it

it into a gally Pot, and take thereof first in the Morning, and last in the Evenings, as much as a good Hasel-nut, with a Spoonful or two of red Wine.

To make a Callice for a Weak Person.

Take a good Chicken, and a Piece of the Neck end of Lamb or Veal, not so much as the Chicken, and set them on the Fire, and when they boil and are well scummed, cast in a large Mace, and the pieces of the bottom of a Manchet, and Half a Handful of French Barly boyled in three Waters before, and put it to the Broth, and take such herbs as the party requireth, and put them in when the Broth hath boiled half an hour, so boil it from three and a half to one; then cast it through a strainer, and scum off all the Fat, so let it cool, then take twenty good Jordan Almonds, or more if they be small, and grind them in a Mortar with some of the Broth, or if you think your broth too strong, grind them with some fair water; and strain them with the Broth; then set it upon a few coals, and season it with some Sugar, not too much, and when it is almost boiled, take out the thickest, and beat it all to pieces in the Mortar, and put it in again, and it will do well, so there be not too much of the others flesh.

For the Gout.

Take six drams of Cariacostine Fasting in the morning, and fast two hours after it, you may roul it up in a Wafer, and take it as Pills, or in Sack, as you conceive is most agreeable for the Stomach; this proportion is sufficient for a Woman, and eight drams for a Man, and take it every second day, until you find remedy for it, it is a gentle Purge that works only upon Winds, and Water.

The Poultess for the Gout.

Take a penny loaf of white bread, and slice it, and put it in fair water, two Eggs beaten together, a handful of red Rose-leaves, two pennyworth of Saffron dryed to powder, then take the Bread out of the Water, and boil it in a quantity of good Milk, with the rest of the Ingredients, and apply it to the place grieved, as warm as you can well endure.

For them that cannot Hear.

Put into their Ears good dryed Suet.

A Sovereign Water good for many Cures, and the health of Bodies.

Take a Gallon of good *Gascoigne* Wine, White, or Claret, then take Ginger, Galingal, Cardomon, Cinnamon, Nutmegs, Grains, Cloves, Annise-seeds, Fennel-seeds, Carraway-seeds, of each of them three drachms; then take Sage, Mints, red Rose-leaves, Thyme, Pellitory, Rosemary, wild Thyme, wild Majoram, Organy, Penni-mountain, Peniroyal, Cammomil, Lavender, Avens, of each of them a handful, then beat the Spices small, and the Herbs, and put all into the Wine, and let it stand for the space of twelve hours, stirring it divers times: then still it in a Limbeck, and keep the first water by it self, for it is best; then will there come a second water, which is good, but not so good as the first: the Virtues of this Water be these. It comforteth the Spirit vital, and preserveth greatly the Spirit vital, and preserveth the youth of man, and helpeth all inward Diseases coming of cold, and against shaking of the Palsie, it cureth the contract of sinews, and helpeth the Conception of the Barren, it killeth the Worms in the Belly, it killeth the Gout, it helpeth Tooth-ach, it comforteth the stomach very much, it cureth the cold Dropsie, it breaketh the Stone in the Back, and in the reins of the Back, it cureth the Canker, it helpeth shortly the stinking Breath, and whosoever useth this water oft, it preserveth them in good liking; this water will be better if it stand

in

in the sun all the Summer, and you must draw of the first water but a pint, and of the second as far as it will run, until the whole Gallon of Wine and Herbs be all done out, but the last water is very small, and not half so good as the first; if you do draw above a pint of the best water, you must have all things more as is aforesaid.

To stanch the bleeding of a Wound.

Take a Hounds-turd, and lay it on a hot coal, and bind it thereto, and that shall stanch bleeding; or else bruise a long worm, and make powder of it, and cast it on the wound; or take the ear of a Hare, and make pouder thereof, and cast that on the Wound, and that will stanch bleeding.

For spitting of blood after a Fall or Bruise.

Take Bittany, Vervain, Nose-bleed, and five-leaved Grass of each a like, and stamp them in a Mortar, and wring out the juice of them, and put to the juice as much goats Milk, and let them seeth together, and let him that is hurt drink of it seven days together, till the waxing of the Moon; and let him drink also Osmory and Cumfrey with stale Ale, and he shall be whole.

For to heal him that spitteth Blood.

Take the juice of Bettany, and temper that with good Milk, and give the sick to drink four days, and he shall be whole.

For to know whether one that hath the Flux shall live or dye.

Take a penny-weight of Trefoile-seed and give him to drink in Wine or Water, and do this three days, and if it cease he shall live, with the help of Medicine, if not, he shall die.

For to stanch the bleeding of a Vein.

Take Rue and seeth it in water, and after stamp it in a Mortar, and lay it on the Vein, then take Lambs-wool that was never washed, and lay that thereon, and that shall stanch bleeding.

For

For a Vein that is evil smitten.

Take Beans and peel away the lack, and seeth them well in Vinegar, and lay them on the Vein hot, in manner of a Plaister.

For one that pisseth Blood.

Take and seeth Garlick in water, till the third part be wasted away, let him drink of the water, and he shall be whole.

For a Woman travelling with Child.

Take and give her Tittany to drink in the morning, and she shall be delivered without peril, or else give her Hysop with water that is hot, and she shall be delivered of the child, although the child be dead and rotten; and anon when she is delivered, give her the same without Wine, or bind the herb Argentine to her Nostrils, and she shall be soon delivered; or else Polipody and stamp it, and lay that on the womans foot in manner of a Plaister, and she shall be delivered quick or dead; or else give her Savory with hot water and she shall be delivered.

Against Surfeiting and Digesting.

Take the bottom of a wheat-loaf, and toast it at the fire, til it be very brown and hard, and then take a good quantity of *Aqua vitæ*, and put upon the same toasted, and put it in a single Linnen cloth, and lay at the breast of the Patient all night, and with the help of God he shall recover, and he shall Vomit or Purge soon after.

A water to comfort weak Eyes, and to preserve the sight.

Take a Gallon and a half of old Wheat, fair and clean picked from all manner of soyle, and then still it in an ordinary Still with a soft fire, and the water that comes of it must be put in a glass, then take half a pound of white sugar candy, and bruise it in a Mortar to pouder, and after three days, when the water hath been in a glass, then put in the powdered Candy; then take an ounce of *Lapis Tutia* tie prepared, and put it into the glass to the rest of the stuff, then take an ounce of Camphire, and break it between your fingers small, and put it into the Glass, then stop the glass close, and the longer it stands, the better it will be.

For tender Eyes, or for Children.

Take a little piece of white Sugar-candy as much as a Chesnut, and put it into three or four spoonfuls of White-wine to steep, then take it out again and dry it, and when it is dry, bruise it in a clean Mortar that tasts of no spice, then put it upon a white Paper, and so hold it to the fire that it may be through dry, and then searce it through a little sieve.

For hot Eyes and red.

Take slugs, such as when you touch them will turn like the pummel of swords, a dozen or sixteen, shake them first in a clean cloth, and then in another, and not wash them, then stamp them, and put three or four spoonfuls of Ale to them, and strain it through a dry cloth, and give it the party morning and evening, first and last.

For Corns.

Take fair water half a pint, Mercury sublimare a penny-worth, Allum as much as a Bean, boil all these together in a Glass Still, till a spoonful be wasted, and always warm it when you use it: this water is also good for any Itch, Tetter, Ring-worm, or Wart.

A Sear-cloth, for a Sore, or Sprain, or any Swelling.

Take Vervain seven ounces, of *Siros* seven ounces, of Camphire three drams, of oyl of Roses ten ounces, let the Wax and the Oil boil till the Wax be melted, then put in your *Siros* finely beaten, stirring it on the fire till it look brown; then put in the Camphire finely beaten, and let it boil two or three walmes, and then dip in your Cloaths.

A Poultess for a Swelling.

Take a good handful of Violet leaves, and as much Groundsel, of Chickweed and Mallowes, half a handful, cut all these with a knife, and so seeth them well in Conduit-water, and thicken it with Barly-meal being finely sifted, and so roul it sure, and lay it to the swelled place, and shift it twice a day.

To make a strong water good for a Canker, or any old Sore, or to eat any lump of flesh that groweth.

Take of Celendine a handful, of red Sage a handful, and of Woodbine-leaves a handful, shred all these together very small, and steep them in a quart of White-wine, and a pint of Water, letting it stand all night, and on the morrow strain it, and put therein of Borax, and Camphire, of each nine penny-worth, and of Mercury four penniworth, and set them on a soft fire; boiling softly for the space of an hour, and when you will use it, warm a little of it, dip in it a cloth, and lay it on the Sore, or dip in it any Cotton.

To heal any Bruise, Sore, or Swelling.

Take two pound of Wax, and two pound of Rosin, and two pound and a half of butter, and four spoonfuls of Flower, and two good spoonfuls of Honey; put in your Wax, Rosin, and your Butter all together, boil all these together, and clarifie it, then put in two ounces of Carmerick, and when it hath thus boiled a quarter of an hour, put a little water in a dish, and put it in, and let it stand till it be cold, and when you will use it, you may melt it on a soft fire, and put in your cloaths, and make Searcloth, and you may spread it Plaister-wise to heal any wound.

A Medicine for any wound old or new.

Take a pint of Sallade Oil, and four ounces of Bees Wax, and two ounces of stone pitch, and two ounces of Rosin, and two ounces of *Venice* Turpentine, and one penny-worth of Frankincense, and a handful of Rosemary tops, and a handful of Tutson leaves, and a handful of Plantain leaves; these herbs must be stamped, and the juice of them put to the things aforesaid, and let them boil together about a quarter of an hour, or thereabouts; this being done, put it into an earthen pot, and when it is cold you may use it as you have occasion, and keep it two year; a most excellent Medicine.

A Medicine for a Wen.

Take black Sope, and unquench Lime, of each alike quantity, beat them very small together, and spread it on a woollen cloth, and lay it on the Wen, and it will consume it away.

For breaking of Childrens heads.

Take of White-wine, and sweet Butter alike, and boil them together till it come to a Salve, and so anoint the head therewith.

For to mundifie, and gently to cleanse Ulcers and breed, new flesh.

Take Rosin eight ounces, *Colophonia* four ounces, *Era. & Oliva, ana.* one pound, *Adypis ovyni, Gum Amoniaci Opoponaci, ana.* one ounce, fine *Eruginis æris*; boil your Wax, *Colophonia*, and Rosin, with the oil together, then strain the Gums, being first dissolved in Vinegar, and boil it with a gentle fire, then take it off, and put in your *Verdigriece*, and fine powder, and use it according to Art.

A Fomentation.

Take the liquor wherein Neats-feet have been boiled, with Butter, and new Milk, and use in manner of a Fomentation.

For the Falling Sickness, or Convulsions.

Take the dung of a Peacock, make it into powder, and give so much of it to the Patient as will lye upon a Shilling, in Succory-water fasting.

For a Tetter, proceeding of a salt humor in the Breast and Paps.

Anoint the sore place with Tanners Owse.

For the Bloody-Flux.

Take the bone of a Gammon of Bacon, and set it up on end in the middle of a Charcoal-fire, and let it burn till it look like Chalk, and that it will burn no longer, then powder it, and give the powder thereof unto the sick.

A Plaster for all manner of Bruises.

Take one pound of Mede Wax, and a quartern of Pitch, half a quartern of Galbanum, and one pound of Sheeps tallow, shred them and seeth them softly, and put them to a little White-wine, or good Vinegar, and take of Frankincense, and Mastick, of each half an ounce in powder, and put it to and boil them all together, and still them till it be well relented, and spread this Salve upon a mighty Canvas that will over-spread the Sore, and lay it thereon hot till it be whole.

To make Flos Unguentorum.

Take Rosin per-rosin, and half a pound of Virgin-wax, Frankincense a quarter of a pound, of Mastick half an ounce, of Sheeps-tallow a quarter of a pound, of Camphire two drams, melt that that is to melt, and powder that that is to powder, and boil it over the fire, and strain it through a cloth into a pottle of White-wine, and boil it all together, and then let it cool a little, and then put thereto a quartern of Turpentine, and stir all well together till it be cold, and keep it well. This Ointment is good for Sores old and new, it suffereth no Corruption in the Wound, nor no evil flesh to be gendered in it, and it is good for headach, and for all manner of Imposthumes in the head, and for Wind in the Brain, and for Imposthumes in the body, and for boiling ears and cheeks, and for sauce flegm in the face, and for Sinews that be be knit or stiff, or sprung with Travel; it doth draw out a thorn, or iron, in what place soever it be, and it is good for the biting or stinging of Venemous Beasts; it rotteth and healeth all manner of Botches without, and it is good for a Fester, and Canker, and *Noli me tangere*, and it draweth out all manner of aking of the Liver, and of the Spleen, and of the Meivis, and it is good for aking and swelling of many Members, and for all Members, and it ceaseth the Flux of Menstrua, and of Emeroids, and it is a special thing to make a fumed cloth to heal all manner of Sores, and it searcheth farthest inward of any Ointment.

An Ointment for all sorts of Aches.

Take Bettone, Cammomile, Celendine, Rosemary, and Rue, of each of them a handful, wash the Herbs, and press out the Water, and then chop or stamp them very small, and then take fresh Butter unwashed and unsalted a quart, and seeth it untill half be wasted, and clarified, then scum it clean, and put in of Oil Olives one ounce, a piece of Virgins-Wax for to harden the Ointment in the Summer time, and if you make it in the Winter, put into your Ointment a little quantity of Foot-Senne instead of the Virgins-Wax.

An excellent Sirrup to purge.

Take of *Scena Alexandrina* one pound, Polipodium of the Oak four ounces, Sarsaparilla two ounces, Damask Prunes four ounces, Ginger seven drams, Annise-seeds one ounce, Cummin-seed half an ounce, Caraway-seeds half an ounce, Cinnamon ten drams, *Aristolchia rotunda*, *Peonia*, of each five drams, Rubarb one ounce, Agarick six drams, Tamarisk two handfuls, boil all these in a gallon of fair Water unto a pottle, and when the Liquor is boiled half away, strain it forth, and then put in your Rubarb and Agarick in a clean thin handkerchief, and tye it up close, and put it

into

into the said Liquor, and then put in two pound of fine Sugar, and boil it to the height of a Sirrup, and take of it the quantity of six spoonfuls, or more or less, as you find it worketh in you.

To make drink for all kind of Surfeits.

Take a quart of *Aqua*, or small *Aqua vitæ*, and put in that a good handful of Cowslip-flowers, Sage-flowers a good handful, & Rosemary-flowers a handful, sweet Marjoram a little, Pellitory of the wall a little, Bettony and Balm, of each a pretty handful, Cinnamon half an ounce, Nutmegs a quarter of an ounce, Fennel-seed, Annise-seed, Coriander-seed, Carraway-seed, Gromwel-seed, Juniper-berries, of each a dram, bruise your Spices and Seeds, and put them into your *Aqua*, or *Aqua vitæ*, with your herbs together, and put to that three quarters of a pound of very fine Sugar; stir them together, and put them in a Glass, and let it stand nine days in the Sun, and let it be stirred every day; it is to be made in *May*, steeped in a wide-mouthed Glass, and strained out into a narrow mouthed Glass.

A Medicine for the Reins of the Back.

Take Housleek, and stamp and strain it, then dip a fine linnen cloth into it, and lay it to the Reins of the Back, and that will heal it.

A Medicine for the Ach in the Back.

Take Egrimony, and Mugwort both leaves and roots, and stamp it with old Bores grease, and temper it with Honey and Eysell, and lay it to the Back.

For a Stitch.

Take Roses, and Cammomil, of each a handful, and oyl of Roses, and oyl of Cammomil, of both together a Saucer full, and a quantity of Barly flower, boil all these together in Milk, and then take a linnen Bag, and put it therein, and lay the Plaister as hot as may be suffered where the Stitch is.

To make a Salve for Wounds that be cankered, and do burn.

Take the juyce of Smallage, of Morrel, of Waberd, of each alike, then take the white of Eggs, and mingle them together, and put thereto a little Wheat-flower, and stir them together till it be thick, but let it come near no fire but all cold; let it be laid on raw to the sore, and it shall cleanse the Wound.

A Medicine for Bone-ach.

Take Brook-lime, and Smallage, and Daisies, with fresh Sheeps-tallow, and fry them together, and make thereof a Plaister, and lay it to the sore hot.

For Sinews that are shrunk.

Take young Swallows out of the Nest a dozen or sixteen, and Rose-mary, Lavender, and rotten Strawberry-leaves, strings and all, of each a handful, after the quantity of the Swallows, the Feathers, Guts and all, bray them in a Mortar, and fry all them together with *May* Butter, not too much; then put it in an Earthen pot, and stop it close nine days: then fry it again with *May* Butter, and fry it well, and strain it well, when you shall use it, chafe it against the fire.

A Water for the biting of a mad Dog.

Take Scabios, Matfiline, Yarrow, Nightshade, wild Sage, the leaves of white Lillies, of each a like quantity, and still them in a common Still, and give the quantity of three or four spoonfuls of the Water mingled with half a handful of Triacle, to any man or beast that is bitten, within three days after the biting, and for lack of the Water take the juices of these Herbs mingled with Triacle, it will keep the sore from rankling; take Dittany, Eg-imony, and rusty Bacon, and beat them fine together, and lay it unto the wound, and it will keep it from rankling.

A proved Medicine for any one that have an Ague in their Breast.

Take the Patients own water, or any others that is very young, and set it on the fire, put therein a good handful of Rosemary, and let it boil; then take two red cloaths, and dip them in the Water, then nip it hard, and lay it on the Breast as hot as it may be endured, and apply it till you see the Breast asswaged, then keep it very warm.

To kill a Fellon.

Take red Sage, white Sope, and bruise them, and lay it to the Fellon, and that will kill it.

To break a Fellon.

Take the grounds of Ale, and as much Vinegar, the crums of leavened Bread, and a little Honey, and boil them all together till they be thick, and lay that hot to the joint where the Fellon is, and that will heal it.

Doctor Stephens Sovereign Water.

Take a gallon of good Gascoign-wine, then take Ginger, Galingal, Cancel, Nutmeg, Grains, Cloves, Annise-seeds, Carraway-seeds, of each a dram; then take Sage, Mint, red Roses, Thyme, Pellitory, Rosemary, wild Thyme, Cammomil, Lavender, of each one handful; then bray both Spices and Herbs, and put them all into the Wine, and let them stand for twelve hours, divers times stirring them; then still that in a Limbeck, but keep that which you still first by it self, for that is the best; but the other is good also, but not so good as the first.

The virtues of this Water are these: It comforteth the Spirits vital, and helpeth the inward Diseases which come of cold; and the shaking of the Palsie; it cureth the contraction of Sinews, and helpeth the conception of Women that be Barren; it killeth worms in the Body; it cureth the cold Cough; it helpeth the Tooth-ach; it comforteth the

the Stomach; it cureth the cold Dropfie; it helpeth the Stone; it cureth shortly the stinking Breath, and who so useth this water enough, but not too much, it preserveh him in good liking, making him young.

Doctor Willoughbies *Water.*

Take Galingal, Cloves, Cubebs, Ginger, Mellilot, Cardamome, Mace, Nutmegs, of each a dram, and of the juice of Celendine half a pint; and mingle all these made in powder with the said juice, and with a pint of good *Aqua vitæ*, and three pints of good White wine, and put all these together in a Still of Glass; and let it stand so all night, and on the morrow still it with an easie fire as may be.

The virtue is of secret nature, it dissolveth the swelling of the Lungs without any grievance, and the same Lungs being wounded or perished, it helpeth and comforteth, and it suffereth not the Blood to putrifie; he shall never need to be let blood that useth this Water, and it suffers not the heart to be burnt, nor melancholly or flegm to have dominion above nature, it also expelleth the Rheum, and purifieth the stomach, it preserveth the visage or memory, and destroyeth the Palsie, and if this water be given to a man or woman labouring towards death, one spoonful relieveth. In the Summer time use once a week fasting the quantity of one spoonful, and in Winter two spoonfuls.

A Medicine for them that have a pain, after their child-bed.

Take Tar, and fresh Barrows grease, and boil it together, then take Pigeons Dung, and fry it in fresh grease, and put it in a bag.

For the drink: Take a pint of Malmsey, and boil it, and put Bay-berries and Sugar in it, the Bay-berries must be of the whitest, and put therein some Sanders.

Take

Take some fair water, and set it over the fire, and put some ground Malt in it, when they use these things they must keep their bed.

For the running of the Reins.

Take *Venice* Turpentine rouled in Sugar and Rose-water, swallow it in pretty roules, and put a piece of Scarlet warm to your back.

For Cods that be swollen.

Stamp Rue and lay thereto.

To draw an Arrow head, or other Iron out of a Wound.

Take the juyce of *Valerian*, in the which you shall wet a Tent, and put it into the wound, and lay the same Herb stamped upon it, then your band or binding as appertaineth, and by this means you shall draw out the Iron, and after heal the Wound as it requireth.

A Plaister for a green Wound.

Take Flower and Milk, and seeth them together till it be thick, then take the white of an Egg and beat them together, and lay it to the Wound, and that will keep it from rankling.

For a Lask.

Take an Egg, and *Aqua vitæ*, and boil it with the Egg till it be dry: then take Cinnamon and Sugar and eat with the Egg.

For him that hath a bunch or knot in his head, or that hath his head swollen with a Fall.

Take one ounce of Bay Salt, raw Honey three ounces, Turpentine two ounces, intermingle all this well upon the fire, then lay it abroad upon a linnen cloth, and thereof make a plaister, the which you shall lay hot to the head, and it will altogether asswage the swelling, and heal it perfectly.

Against the biting of any venemous Beast.

As soon as the person feeleth himself bit with any venemous beast, or at least, so soon as it is possible, let him take green leaves of Fig-tree, and press the Milk of them three or four times into the wound:

And

And for this also serveth Mustard-seed mingled with Vinegar.

A perfect Remedy for him that is sore wounded with any Sword or Staff.

Take *Taxas barbatus*, and stamp it, and take the juyce of it, and if the Wound bleed, wipe it, and make it clean, washing it with White-wine, or Water, then lay the said juices upon the wound, and the herb whereof you take the juyce, upon it, then make your band, and let it abide on a whole day, and you shall see a wonderful effect.

A Bag to smell unto for Melancholy, or cause one to sleep.

Take dry Rose leaves, keep them close in a glass which will keep them sweet, then take powder of Mints, powder of Cloves in a gross powder, and put the same to the Rose-leaves, then put all these together in a bag, and take that to bed with you, it will cause you to sleep, it is good to smell unto at other times.

For spitting of Blood.

Take the juice of Bettony tempered with Goats Milk, and drink thereof three or four mornings together.

An Ointment for all Sores, Cuts, Swellings, and Heat.

Take a good quantity of Smallage, and Mallowes, and put thereto two pound of Bores grease, one pound of Butter, and oil of Neats-foot a quantity, stamp them well together, then fry them, and strain them into an earthen pot, and keep it for your use.

A Salve for a New Hurt.

Take the whitest Virgins wax you can get, and melt it in a pan, then put in a quantity of Butter and Honey, and seeth them together, then strain them into a dish of fair water, and work it in your Hands, and make it in a round Ball, and so keep it, and when you will use it, work some of it between your Hands, strike it upon a cloth, and

and lay it upon the Sore, and it will draw and heal it.

Against the biting of a Mad Dog, and the Rage or Madness that followeth a Man after he is Bitten.

Take the blossomes or flowers of wild Thistles dried in the shade, and beaten to powder, give him to drink of that powder in white Wine half a Walnut shell full, and in thrice taking it he shall be healed.

Against spitting of Blood by reason of some Vein broken in the Breast.

Take Mise dung beaten into powder, as much as will lye upon a groat, and put it in half a glass full of the juice of Plantane with a little sugar, and so give the Patient to drink thereof in the morning before breakfast, and at night before he go to bed, continuing the same, it will make him whole and sound.

For to cleanse the Head.

Take Pellitory of *Spain*, and chew the roots three days, a good quantity, and it will purge the head, and do away the Ach, and fasten the teeth in the gums.

A good Remedy against the Plurisie.

Open a white loaf in the middle new baked, and spread it well with Triacle on both the halfs on the crown side, and heat it at the fire, then lay one of the halfs on the place of the disease, and the other half on the other side of the body directly against it, and so bind them that they loose not, nor stir, leaving them so a day and a night, or until the Imposthume break, which I have sometimes seen in two hours or less, then take away the bread, and immediately the Patient will begin to spit and void the putrefaction of the Imposthume, and after he hath slept a little, you shall give him meat, and with the help of God he shall shortly heal.

Rare Secrets in Physick.

For a Pin, or Web in the Eye.

Take two or three Lice out of ones head, and put them alive into the eye that is grieved and so close it up, and most assuredly the Lice will suck out the Web in the eye, and will cure it, and come forth without any hurt.

A Remedy to be used in a fit of the Stone when the water stops.

Take the fresh shells of Snails, the newest will look of a reddish colour, and are best, take out the Snails, and dry the shells with a moderate heat in an oven after the bread is drawn, likewise take Bees and dry them so, and beat them severally into powder, then take twice so much of the Bees powder as the Snails, and mix them well together, keep it close covered in a glass, and when you use it, take as much of this powder as will lie upon a sixpence, and put it into a quarter of a pint of the distilled water of Bean-flowers, and drink it fasting, or upon an empty stomach, and eat nor drink nothing, for two or three hours after.

This is good to cause the party to make urine, and bring away the gravel or stone that causeth the stopping, and hath done very much good.

A Sirrup for the pain in the Stomach.

Take two good handfuls of young Rue, boil it in a quart of good White-wine Vinegar till it be half consumed, so soon as it is through cold, strain it, and put to every pint of the liquor a pound and and a quarter of Loaf-sugar, and boil it till it come to a Sirrup, when you use it, take a good spoonful of this in the morning fasting, and eat nor drink nothing for two or three hours after; it is good for pain in the stomach that proceeds from windy vapours, and is excellent good for the Lungs and obstructions of the Breast.

Receipts for bruises, approved by the Lady of Arundel.

Take black Jet, beat it to powder, and let the patient

patient drink it every morning in beer till it be well.

Another for the same.

Take the sprigs of Oak-trees, and put them in a paper, rost them, and break them, and drink as much of the powder as will lye upon a sixpence every morning, until the Patient be well.

To cause easie labour.

Take ten or twelve days before her looking, six ounces of brown Sugar-candy beaten to powder, a quarter of a pound of Raisins of the Sun stoned, two ounces of Dates unstoned sliced, half an ounce of Annise-seeds bruised, a quarter of an ounce of Cowslip flowers, one dram of Rosemary flowers, put these in a fine lawn bag with a flint stone, that it may sink into a pottle of White-wine, let it steep 24 hours, and after take of it in the morning, and at four in the afternoon, and in the evening, the quantity of a wine glass full.

A Cordial for the Sea.

Take one ounce of Sirrup of Clove-Gilliflowers, one dram of *Confectio Alchermes*, one ounce and a half of Borrage-water, and the like of Mint-water, one ounce of Mr. *Mountfords* water, and as much of Cinnamon water, temper all these together in a Cordial, and take a spoonful at a time when you are at Sea.

A Plaister to strengthen the Back.

Take eight yolks of Eggs new laid, one ounce of Frankincense beaten into fine powder, mingle them well together, put in as much Barly flower as will make it thick for a Plaister, spread it on leather, lay it to the small of the back, letting it lye nine hours, use four plaisters one after another, you must slit the plaister in the midst, so as it may not lye on the back bone.

A present Remedy for a Woman with child that hath taken harm by fall, or fright, or any mischance.

To stay the Child, and strengthen it, take one ounce of Pickerel jaws, fine beaten and searced, of Dates stones, and *Bole armoniack*, of each one ounce, of *Sanguis Draconis*, half an ounce, give of these, being well searced and mingled together, a French Crown weight in Musk dine or Malmsey, and let the woman keep her very warm.

For a weak Back

Take of red Lead half a pound, of white Lead half a pound, boil these in three pints of Sallade oil in a pipkin, stirring them continually with a piece of Iron, until it be of a grey colour, then roul it up in roules, and keep it for your use.

Oil of Saint Johns Wort

Take a quart of Sallade oil, put thereto a quart of the flowers of St. *Johns* Wort well picked, let them lye therein all the year till the Seeds be ripe, the glass must be kept warm, either in the Sun or in water all the Summer until the seeds be ripe, then put in a quarter of St. *Johns* Wort seeds whole, and so let it stand twelve hours, then you must seeth the oil eight hours, the glass being kept open, and the water in the pot full as high as the oil is of height in the glass; then when it is cold strain it, that the seeds may not remain in the oil, and then put up the oil for your use.

A green Salve for an old Sore.

Take a handful of Groundsel, as much Housleek, of Marigold leaves a handful, pick and wipe these Herbs clean, but wash them not, then beat all these Herbs in a wooden bowl as small as is possible, then strain out all the juice, and put in a quantity of Hogs grease, as much as two Eggs, beat all these together again, then put in the juice again, and put in ten Eggs, yolks and whites, five spoonfuls of English Honey, and as much Wheat flower as will make all this as thick as a salve, and so stir it very well together, and put it close up in a pot that it take no air, and so keep it for your use.

A most excellent Powder for the Cholick and Stone.

You must take it morning and evening before you go to bed, *Sperma Cœti* one ounce and half, Cloves and Mace one quarter of an ounce, Anniseeds and *Per stone*, of each two ounces, Cinnamon, and small Pepper, of each one quarter of an ounce, Date-stones a quarter of an ounce, Liquorice, Fennel, red Sage, Bay-berries, of each three quarters of an ounce, Acorns one quarter and half of an ounce, Lilly roots two drams, the white of Oyster shells burned in the fire, one quarter of an ounce; beat all these into fine powder, and drink as much thereof in Ale or Beer as will lie on a sixpence, and fast one hour or two after it: If the party before grieved take one handful of Parsly, and seeth it in Ale until half be sod away, with twenty or thirty Prunes therein strained, and put thereto two spoonfuls of this powder, and drink it mornings and evenings, somewhat warm.

A present Remedy for the running of the Reins.

Take an ounce of Nutmegs, half an ounce of Mastick, then slice the Nutmegs, and put them in steep in Rose Vinegar all one night, then lay them in a dish to dry before the fire, then take the Mastick and lay it in Papers, and beat it with a hammer very small, and put a little Corral well beaten unto it, and as much Ambergriece, then mingle these things together with Sugar, and make it pleasant to eat, and so take a good quantity morning and evening.

A Salve for a green Wound.

Take two handfuls of Water-dittany, two handfuls of Rosemary shred very small, a quarter of a pint of Turpentine, half a pound of yellow Wax, a quart of Sallade oil, half a pint of White-wine,

boil

boil all these together while the White-wine be quite consumed, then it will be green and come to the height of a Salve.

A proved Medicine for a burning or scalding, by lightning or otherwise.

Take Hogs greafe, or Sheeps treacles, and Alehoof, beat these very well together, then take more Hogs greafe, and boil it to a Salve.

To use it.

Anoint the place grieved with this Ointment, and then lay upon the sore so anointed Colewart leaves, which must be boiled very soft in water, and the strings made smooth with beating them with a Pestle.

A Powder for the green Sickness, approved with very good success upon many.

Take of Cloves, Mace, Nutmegs, of each one quarter of an ounce, beat them severally, and then altogether very well, fine sugar very small beaten one quarter of a pound, and then mix and beat them all four together; Pearl the sixth part of half an ounce finely beaten, mingle it with the rest, and beat them all together again, the filing of Steel or Iron an ounce and a quarter, sift it very fine, and mingle it with the rest, but if so small a quantity will not serve, add a quarter more of the mettal, let it be sifted before you weigh it, but if all this will not serve the turn, put in a little Rubarb, or a little Aloe-succarrina.

The Manner of using this Powder.

In the morning when you rise take half a spoonful of it, as much at four a clock in the afternoon, and as much, when you go to bed, walk or stir much after the first taking of it, I mean every morning and evening, fast one hour after the taking of it, or more, and then eat some Sugarsops or thin Broth.

The Patients Diet.

She must forbear Oatmeal in broth or any other thing, Cheese, Eggs, Custards, or any stopping Meat, take care that this be not given to any Woman that hath conceived or is with Child.

A Drink to stanch Blood Inwardly.

Take the Juyce of one handful of Shepheards purse, of Parsley, and Five-finger, of each as much, take five slips of Egrimony, strain all these juyces into the Milk of a red Cow, and drink thereof early and late warm.

A Powder to keep the Teeth clean, and from Worm-eaten.

Take Rosemary burned to Ashes, Cuttles-bone, Harts-horn burned to powder, Sal gemmæ, twelve penny weight, the flowers of Pomegranates, white Coral, of each a six-penny weight, make all these in powder, and with a little Rose-water, and a Sage Leaf, rub the Teeth.

A Salve to Heal all manner of Sores and Cuts.

Take one pint of Turpentine, one pint of oil Olive, a quarter of a pint of running Water, nine branches of Rosemary, one ounce of unwrought Wax, two ounces of Rosat, seeth all these together in a little pan over the Fire, let it seeth until there arise a little white scum upon it, then stir it with a stick, suffering it to boil until one quarter be consumed, then take it from the Fire, strain it through a course cloth, but it must be done quickly after it be taken from the fire for cooling, after you have strained it into an earthen pot, let it cool, and keep it for your use.

To make Oil of Sage, good for the Grief in any Joynt, or for any Ach.

Take Sage and Parsly, seeth them in the oil Olive, till it be thick and green.

A Medicine to Purge and Amend the Heart, Stomach, Spleen, Liver, Lungs, and Brain.

Take Alexander, Water-cresses, young Mallows, Bor-

Borrage, and Fennel Roots pared, Mercury, Hartstongue, and Clare, and make of these Pottage.

To drive infectious Diseases from the Heart.

Take Mithridate, and Century, of each two ounces, eight spoonfuls of Dragon Water, one pint of white Wine, seven spoonfuls of *Aqua vitæ*, boil all together a little, strain it, then set it on the Fire again a little while, and drink of it morning and evening.

For the Tooth-ach.

Take Pepper and Grains, of each one ounce, bruise them, and compound them with the water of the diseased, and make it of a good thickness, and lay it outward on the Cheek against the place grieved, and it will help it for ever after.

Another.

Take dryed Sage, make powder of it, burnt Allum, Bay Salt dryed, make all in fine powder, and lay it to the Tooth where the pain is, and also rub the Gums with it.

For the Strangullion or the Stone.

Take the inner rind of a Young Ash, between two or three Years of Growth, dry it to powder, and drink of it as much at once, as will lie on a Sixpence in Ale or white Wine, and it will bring present Remedy: The Party must be kept Warm two hours after it.

For the Stone.

Take the Stone that groweth within the gall of an Ox, grate it, and drink of it in white Wine, as much as will lie upon a Sixpence at once, for want of white Wine make a Posset of Ale, and clarifie the Ale from the Curd, then boil one handful of Pellitory therein, and drink of the powder with it.

For the Black-Jaundies.

Take Earth Worms, wash them in white Wine, then dry them, and beat them into powder, and put to a little Saffron, and drink it in Beer.

A drawing Salve for an old Sore.

Take Rosin half a pound beaten to powder, Sheeps Tallow a quarter of a pound, melt them together, and pour them into a Bason of Water, and when they begin to cool a little, work them well with your Hands in the Water, and out of the Water, drawing it up and down the space of one hour till it be very white, then make it up in Rouls, and reserve it, to strike thin Plaister upon old Sores.

A Water to Wash Sores withal.

Take Wormwood, Sage, Plantain Leaves, of each one Handful, Allum two ounces, Hony two Saucers full, boil all these together in three pints of Water till half be consumed, then strain it, and reserve that Liquor to wash the Sore withal.

A Medicine to Cure the Garget in the Throat.

Take a pint of May Butter, and put it on the Fire in a Posnet, and put into it of the inner bark of Elder one good handful, and some Daisie Roots, seeth it to half the Quantity, and strain it, and so keep it cool; take this Ointment and Anoint your Throat, then take the Ointment, and strike a long Plaister with it very thick of the Ointment, then strike upon the Ointment the best Jane Triacle, and upon that strew grosse Pepper very thick, strike it on with a Knife, Warm the Plaister, and bind it round your Throat to your Ears, renew it once a Day with the Ointment, and the Triacle, and Pepper, and lay it on again, before you use this Ointment, scour your Mouth and Throat with the powder of Roch Allum burned, mix it with the powder of Madder or Pepper.

For the Hearing.

Take an Onion, take the Core out of it, fill it with Pepper, slice it in the midst, being first wrapt in Paper and roasted in the Embers, lay it to each Ear.

For a Dead Child in a Womans Body.

Take the juyce of Hyſop, temper it in Warm Water, and give it the Woman to Drink.

For a Woman that hath her Flowers too much.

Take a Hares Foot and burn it, make powder of it, and let her drink it with ſtale Ale.

A Medicine for the Gout.

Take Tetberry Roots, waſh and ſcrape them Clean, and ſlice them Thin, then take the Greaſe of a Barrow Hog, the Quantity of either alike, then take an earthen pot, then lay a lain of Greaſe in the bottom, then a lain of Roots, then the Greaſe again, and ſo Roots and Greaſe till the pot be full, then ſtop the pot very cloſe, and ſet it in a Dung-hil one and Twenty Days, then beat it altogether in a boul, then boil it a good while, then ſtrain it, and put in a penni-worth of *Aqua vitæ*, then Anoint the Place grieved very Warm againſt the Fire.

A Diet Drink for the running Gout, ach in the Joynts, and for all Infections.

Set ſeven quarts of Water on the Fire, and when it boileth put therein four ounces of *Sarſaparilla* bruiſed, and let it boil two hours very ſoftly, cloſe ſtopped or covered, then put in four ounces of Sene, three ounces of Liquorice bruiſed, of *Stæcados Hermodactil, Epithymum*, and of Cammomil flowers, of every one half an ounce, and ſo boil all theſe two hours very ſoftly, then ſtrain it, and keep it in a cloſe Veſſel cloſe ſtopped, when it is cold, then boil again all the aforeſaid Ingredients in ſeven quarts of Water four hours, with a ſoft Fire cloſe covered; then ſtrain it and keep it as the other by it ſelf, and take of the firſt a good draught one hour before you ariſe in the morning, and a draught at the beginning of Dinner, and another at Supper, and going to Bed, and at all other times; drink of the latter when you liſt, and Eat no Meat but dry roaſted Mutton, Capon,

Rab-

Rabbot, without Salt, and not basted, but to your Breakfast, a poached Egg, no Bread but Bisket, or dryed Crust, and at night Raisins of the Sun, and Bisket-bread; drink no other Drink but this.

A Plaister to Heal any Sore.

Take of Sage, Herb-grace, of each a like quantity, Ribwort, Plaintain, and Daisie Roots, more than half so much of each of them, with Wax, fresh Grease, and Rosin make it a Salve; if the Flesh grow proud, then put always upon the Plaister before you lay it to the Sore, burnt Allum, and it will correct the Flesh.

To cause a Woman to have her Sickness.

Take Egrimony, Motherwort, Avens and Parsley, shred them small with Oatmeal; make Pottage of them with Pork; let her eat the Pottage, but not the Pork.

For the Stone

Take the green Weed of the Sea, which is brought with Oisters, wash it, and dry it to powder, Drink it with Malmsey Fasting.

To Kill Worms.

Take Aloe succatrina two ounces, let it stand in a quart of Malmsey eight hours; drink it morning and evening.

For a Hot Rheum in the Head.

Take Rose-water, Vinegar, and Sallade-oil, mix them well together, and lay it to the Head Warm.

For a Lask.

Take the nether Jaw of a Pike, beat it to powder and drink it.

For an Itch or any Scurf of the Body

Take Elecampane-roots, or Leaves, stamp them; and fry them with fresh Grease, strain it into a dish, and Anoint the Patient.

For one that is bruised with a Fall.

Take Horse-dung, and Sheeps suet, boil them together, and apply it to the same place, being laid upon a cloth.

For the *Emerhoides*.

Take Hops and Vinegar, fry them together, and put it into a little bag, and lay it as Hot as may be endured to the Fundament, divers bags one after another, and let one continue at it.

For one that is burned with Gunpowder, or otherwise.

Take one handful of Groundsel, twelve heads of Houfleek, one pint of Goose-dung, as much Chickens-dung, of the newest that may be gotten, stamp the Herbs as small as you can, then put the dung into a Mortar, temper them together with a pottle of Bores-grease, labour them together half an hour, and strain it through a Canvas bag with a cleft stick into an earthen pan, and use it when need requireth, it will last two Year.

To Heal a Prick with a Nail or Thorn.

Take two handfuls of Celendine, as much Orpen, cut it small, and boil it with Oil-olive, and unwrought Wax, then strain it, and use it.

To stop the Bleeding of a Cut or Wound.

Take Hop, stamp it, and put it into the Wound, if Hop will not do it, then put to it Vinegar with the Hop.

For a *Scald*.

Take the Leaves of ground Ivie, three handfuls, Houfleek one handful, wash them and stamp them in a stone Mortar very small, and as you stamp them, put in a pint of Cream by little and little; then strain it, and put it in a pot with a Feather, take of this and Anoint the scalded place, and then wet a Linnen cloth in the same Ointment; and lay it on the place; and over that roul other Cloths.

An Ointment for a Tetter.

Take *Salarmoniack* one ounce, beat it into fine powder, then mix it with Sope and fresh Grease, of each two ounces; make an Ointment and Anoint the Place.

For the Singing in the Head.

Take one Onion, cut out the core, and fill that place with the pouder of Cummin, and the juice of Rue, set on the top again, and roast the Onion in embers; then put away the outside, and put it in a cloth, wring out the juice; take black Wool and dip it in, put this into thine ear where the singing is, and if it be on both sides, then serve one after another.

A Drink for one that is Weak, and misdoubting a Consumption.

Take three handfuls of Rosemary, bruise it a little, and close it in paste, bake it in an Oven until it be well dryed, then cut the paste and take forth the Rosemary: infuse it in two quarts of Claret-wine, with two ounces of good Triacle, one ounce of Nutmegs, of Cinnamon, and Ginger, of each half an ounce bruised; let them stand infused two nights and one day, then distil it in a Limbeck; drink hereof one spoonful or two next your heart.

A Drink for the Plague.

Take red Sage, Herb-grace, Elder-leaves, red Briar-leaves, of each one handful, stamp them and strain them with a quart of White-wine, and then put to it *Aqua vitæ* and Ginger; drink hereof every morning one spoonful nine mornings together, and it will preserve you.

For a Bruise or Stitch.

Take the Kernels of Walnuts, and small Nuts, Figs, Rue, of each one handful, white Salt the quantity of one Walnut, one race of Ginger, one spoonful of Hony; beat them all together very fine, and eat of it three or four times every Day; make a Plaister of it, and lay it to the place grieved.

A Drink for one that hath a Rupture.

Take Comfrey one good handful, wild Daisie-roots as much, and the like of knotted Grass; stamp all these together, and strain it with Malmsey, fey, and give it to the Patient to drink morning and evening, nine days blood-warm. If it be a Man that hath been long so, he must lye nine days upon his back, and stir as little as he can. If he be a Child, he must be kept so much lying as you may for nine days; if you think the drink too strong for the Child, give it him but five days in Malmsey, and the rest in stale Ale; have a care that the party have a good Truss, and keep him trussed one whole year at the least.

Against the Grief in the Lungs, and Spitting of Blood.

Take the Herb called of the Apothecary *Ungula Caballina*, in English, Colts-foot, incorporated well with the lard of a Hog chopped, and a new laid Egg, Boil it together in a Pan, and give it to the Patient to eat; doing this nine mornings, you shall see a marvellous thing; this is also good to make a Man Fat.

A Plaister for a Rupture.

Take the juyce of Comfrey, wild Daisie-roots, and knotted Grass, of each a like quantity, fresh Butter, and unwrought Wax, of each a like quantity, clarifie them severally, then take of the roots of Comfrey, dry it and make pouder of it; take the powder of Annise-seed, and Cummin-seed, but twice as much Cummin-seed as Annise-seed; boil these pouders in the Butter, and unwrought Wax on a soft fire a good while, then put in your juyce, let it boil a walm or two, so take it from the fire, stir it all together till it be cold; take hereof and spread it, and lay it to his Cods as hot as he can suffer it, and use this till he be whole; this plaister is most excellent for a Child that is burst at the Navil.

GRATIOSA CURA.

A Water for a Cut or Sore.

Take Honeysuckles the knots ript off, flowers of Celendine, flowers of red Sage, of each three spoonfuls, Five-finger, Comfrey such as is to knit bones, Daisies with the roots thereon, Ladder of Heaven, blossoms of Rosemary, Setwel, Herb-grace, Smallage, red Roses with the knots on, or else red Rose-cakes, Adders-tongue, of each of these one handful; seeth all together in six gallons of Water that runneth towards the East, until two gallons be sod in; then strain them, and put to the water three quarts of *English* Honey, one pound of Roach-Allum, one penniworth of Madder, one penniworth of long Pepper, seeth all together until one gallon be consumed; then cleanse the Water.

For the Wind-Collick.

Take the flowers of Walnuts, and dry them to powder, and take of them in your Ale, or Beer, or in your Broth as you like best, and it will help you.

To make a soveraign Oil of a Fox, for the nummed Palsie.

Take a Fox new killed, cased, and bowelled, then put into the body, of Dill, Mugwort, Cammomil, Campits, Southernwood, red Sage, Origanum, Hop, *Stæcad*, Rosemary, Costmary, Cowslip-flowers, Balm, Bettony, sweet Marjoram, of each a good handful, chop them small, and put thereto of the best Oil of Castor, Dill, and Cammomil, of each four ounces: mix the Hearbs and Oils together, and strow over them *Aphronitum* a good handful; put them all into the Fox, and sew up his belly close, and with a quick fire rost him, and the Oil that droppeth out is a most singular Oil for all Palsies or numness. Approved.

To comfort the Brain, and procure Sleep.

Take brown bread crums, the quantity of one Walnut, one Nutmeg beaten to powder, one dram of Cinnamon; put these into a Napkin, with two spoonfuls of Vinegar, four Spoonfuls of Rosewater, and one of Womans Milk.

For the weakness in the Back.

Take the pith of an Ox back, put it into a pottle of Water; then seeth it to a quart, then take a handful of Comfrey, one handful of knotted grass, one hand-

handful of Sheepherds Purse; put these into a quart of Water; boil them unto a pint, with six Dates boiled therein.

For a Canker in any part of the Body.

Take Filberd, Nut-leaves, Lavender Cotton, Southerwood, Worm-wood, Sage, Woodbine-leaves, Sweet Bryar-leaves, of each a like Quantity, of Allum and Hony a good Quantity; seeth all these till they be half sodden, wash the Sore with it.

For an Old Bruise.

Take one spoonful of the juyce of Tansie, and as much Nip, two Pennyworth of *Sperma Ceti*; put it into a little Ale, and drink it.

Oil of Foxes, or Badgers, for Ach in the Joynts, the Sciatica, Diseases of the Sinews, and Pains of the Reins and Back.

Take a Live Fox or Badger, of a middle Age, of a full Body, well Fed, and Fat, Kill him, Bowel and Skin him; some take not out his Bowels, but only his Excrements in his Guts, because his Guts have much Grease about them; Break his Bones small, that you may have all the Marrow; this done, set him a boiling in Salt Brine, and Sea-water, and Salt-water of each a pint and half; of Oil three pints, of Salt three ounces; in the end of the Decoction put thereto the Leaves of Sage, Rosemary, Dill, Organy, Marjoram, and Juniper-berries: And when he is so sodden that his Bones and Flesh do part in sunder, strain all through a strainer, and keep it in a Vessel to make Lineaments for the Ach in the joynts, the Sciatica, Diseases of the Sinews, and Pains of the Reins and Back.

To make the Leaden Plaister.

Take two pound and four ounces of oil Olive of the best, of good red Lead one pound, white Lead one pound well beaten to Dust, twelve ounces of Spanish Sope: And incorporate all these well together in an Earthen pot well glazed before you put them to boil, and when they are well incorporated that the Sope cometh upward, put it upon a small Fire of Coals, continuing the Fire for the space of one hour and a half, still stirring it with an Iron-ball upon the end of a Stick; then make the Fire somewhat bigger, until the redness be turned into a gray Colour, but you must not leave stirring till the matter be turned into the colour of Oil, or somewhat darker, then drop of it upon a Wooden Trencher, and if it cleave not to the Finger it is enough, then make it up into Rouls, it will keep Twenty Years, the older the better.

The Virtue of the Plaister.

The same being laid upon the Stomach, provoketh Appetite, it taketh away any Grief in the Stomach, being laid on the Belly is a present Remedy for the Cholick, and laid unto the Reins of the Back; it is good for the Bloody Flux, running of the Reins, the heat of the Kidneys, and weakness of the Back; the same healeth all Swellings, Bruises, and taketh away Ach; it breaks Felons, Pushes, and other Imposthumes, and healeth them; the same draweth out any running Humour, without breaking the Skin, and being applyed to the Fundament, it Healeth any Disease there Growing; being laid on the Head is good for the Uvula, it helpeth the Head-ach, and is good for the Eyes.

For a Pricking of a Thorn.

Take fine Wheat flower boulted Temper it with Wine, and seeth it thick, lay it hot to the Sore.

A Medicine for the Plague.

Take a pint of Malmsey, and burn it well, then take about six spoonfuls thereof, and put to the quantity of a Nutmeg of good Treacle, and so much Spice Grains beaten as you can take up with the tops of your two Fingers; mix it together, and
let

let the Party Sick drink it Blood-warm; if he be infected it will procure him to cast, which if he do, give him as much more, and so still again and again, observing still some Quantity till the Party leave casting, and so after he will be well, if he cast not at all, once taking it is enough, and probably it is not the Sickness, after the Party hath let casting, it is good to take a competent draught of burnt Malmsie alone with Treacle and Grains; it will Comfort much.

Another Medicine for the Plague.

Take of Setwel grated one Root, of Jane Triacle two spoonfuls, of Wine Vinegar Three spoonfuls, of fair Water three spoonfuls, make all these more than Luke-warm, and drink them off at once well steeped together, Sweat after this six or seven hours, and it will bring forth the Plague-sore.

To break the Plague Sore.

Lay a roasted Onion, all seeth a white Lilly-root in Milk, till it be as thick as a Poultess, and lay it to the same, if these fail, launce the Sore, and so draw it and heal it with Salves for Botches or Biles.

To make a Salve to Dress any Wound.

Take Rosin and Wax, of each half a Pound, of Deer Suet, and Frankincense, of each one quarter of a pound; of Mastick in powder one ounce; boil all these in a pint of White-wine half an hour with a soft Fire, and stir it in the boiling that it run not over; then take it from the Fire, and put thereto half an ounce of Camphire in powder, when it is almost cold, put thereto one quarter of a pound of Turpentine; after all these be mingled together, then put it into the White-wine, and wash it as you wash Butter, and then as it cools make it up in Rouls.

A most Excellent Water for Sore Eyes.

Take a quart of Spring-water, set it upon the Fire in an Earthen Pipkin; then put into it three spoonfuls of white Salt, and one spoonful of white Coperas, then boil them a quarter of an hour, scum it as it doth boil; then strain it through a fine Linnen Cloath, and keep it for your use.

When you take it you must lye down upon the Bed, and drop two drops of it into your Eye, so rest one quarter of an hour, not wiping your Eyes, and use it as often as need shall require.

If the Eye have any Pearl or Film growing upon it; then take a handful of red double Daisie-leaves, and stamp them, and strain them through a linnen cloath, and drop thereof one drop into your Eye, using it three times

A Plaister for one that is bruised.

Take half a pint of Sallade Oil, or Neats-foot-Oil, half a pint of English Hony, two or three perny-worth of Turpentine, a good quantity of Hogs greafe, two or three penny-worth of *Bole Armoniack*, half a pint of strong Wine Vinegar, half a dozen of Egshels, and all beaten very small, one handful of white Salt; put all these together into an Earthen pot, stir and mingle them together exceeding well, then as much Bean-flower, or Wheat-flower, as will thicken it plaisterwise; then with your hand strike it on the grieved place once a Day, and by Gods help it will ease any fore that cometh by means of striking, wrinching, bruising, or other kind of swelling that proceedeth of evil Humours.

Balm-water for a Surfeit.

Take two gallons of strong Ale, and one quart of Sack; take four pound of young Balm-leaves, and shred them; then take one pound of Annise-feeds, and as much Liquorice beaten to powder; put them all into the Ale and Sack to steep twelve hours; put it into a Limbeck, and so still it; it is good for a Surfeit of choller, for to Comfort the heart, and for an Ague.

A Restorative Water in sickness, the Patient being weak.

Take three pints of very good new Milk, and put thereto one pint of very good red Wine, the yolks of twenty one Eggs, and beat them together, that done, put in as much fine Manchet as shall suck up the Milk and Wine; then put the same into a fair Stillatory, and still it with a soaking fire: and take a spoonful of this Water in your Pottage or Drink, and this in one or two months will prevent the Consumption.

To make a Caudle to prevent the Lask.

Take half a pound of unblanched Almonds, stamp them, and strain it into a quart of Ale, and set it on the fire; then take the yolks of four Eggs, and make it for a Caudle, and so season it with a good quantity of Cinnamon and Sugar, and eat it every morning at breakfast.

For one that cannot make water, and to break the Stone.

Pare a Raddish root, and slice it then, and put it into a pint of White-wine, and let it infuse six or seven hours, then strain it, and set it on the fire; and put thereto one Parsley root, and one spoonful of Parsley seed, and half a handful of Pellitory of the wall, and seeth it until half be wasted, and give it luke-warm to drink.

The Diet against Melancholly.

Take Sene eight ounces, Rubarb six drams, Polipody of the Oak, *Sarsaparilla*, and Madder roots, of each four ounces, Annise-seeds, Fennel-seeds, *Epithymum*, of each one ounce, Mace, Cloves, and Nutmegs, of each two ounces, Egrimony, Scabios, and red Dock roots of each one handful, make them all small, and put it into a long narrow bag or boulter, hang it in a vessel of Ale that containeth six gallons, when it is a week old, drink it morning and evening for the space of one fortnight, keep you all that time warm, and a good diet.

A Sirrup to open the Liver.

Take Lungwort, Maidenhair, Egrymony, Scabios, of each one handful, Champitis, Hysop of each a dozen Crops, Endive, and Succory, of each three or four leaves, of young Fennel and Parsley, of each one root, one stick of Liquorice, one spoonful of Barberries clean washed, one spoonful of Annifeseeds, twenty Raisins of the Sun stoned; boil all these in a pottle of water to a quart, then strain it, and put thereto of the best Sugar one quarter of a pound, Conserve of Violets one ounce, and so boil it as long as any scum ariseth, then strain it again, and use this very warm.

For one that cannot make water.

Take the seeds of parsley, of red Fennel, of Saxifrage, of Carraways, of the kernel of Hip-berries, of each a like quantity, put in some pouder of Jet, mingle these, being beaten to pouder, well together, and drink it in stale Ale luke-warm.

To make Aqua Composita.

Take of Annise seeds and Liquorice bruised, of each half a pound. Thyme, and Fennel, of each half a handful, Calamint two handfuls, Coriander, and Carraway seeds bruised of each two ounces, Rosemary, and Sage of each half a handful, infuse these a whole night in three gallons of red Wine, or strong Ale, then still it in a Limbeck with a soft fire.

An Ointment for a Swelling.

Take of Marsh Mallowes, of Wormwood, of Smallage, of each one handful, boil it with one pound of the grease of a Barrow Hog, until it be very green, then strain it and keep it very close. Lady *Pawlet.*

A Plaister for the Back.

Take half a pint of Oil of Roses, four ounces of white Lead ground into fine powder, put your

Oil into a clean Posnet, and set it on the fire, and when it is warm, put in your white Lead, ever stirring it, then put into it of your Wax one quarter, stir it until it be black, then take it from the fire, and in the cooling put thereto two penniworth of Camphire, of white Sanders, and yellow Sanders, of each the weight of four pence, fine *Bole*, and *Terra sigillata*, of each two penny weight, in fine powder all, still stirring it till it be almost cold, and so make it up in rouls: use it as need requires for all weakness, wasting, or heat in the Kidneys. *Cramsh.*

To make Oyl of Swallows.

Take one handful of Mother Thyme, of Lavender-cotton, and Strawberry-leaves, of each alike, four Swallows, feathers and all together well bruised, three ounces of Sallade Oil, beat the Herbs and the Swallows, feathers, and all together, until they be so small that you can see no feathers, then put in the Oil, and stir them well together, and seeth them in a posnet, and strain them through a canvas cloth, and so keep it for your use.

For a Thorn, Fellon, or Prick.

Take the juyce of Fetherfew, of Smallage, of each one saucer full, put to it as much of Wheatflower, as will make it somewhat thick, and put to it of good black Sope the quantity of a Walnut, mingle them together, and lay them to the Sore.

A Drink for one that hath a Rupture.

Take the Comfit, otherwise called Bonesel, a pretty handful, of Woodbitten as much, Bread, Plantain, and leaves of Cammock, somewhat more than a handful, of Vervin as much as of the Cammock, of Daisie roots a small quantity, of Elder tops, or young buds, the least quantity, stamp all these together and put unto them, being stamped, one pint of pure White-wine, then strain it and drink of it morning and evening, one hour or more before

before Breakfast or Supper, a good draught blood-warm.

If it be a sucking Child, let the Nurse drink posset-ale of the aforesaid drink, and let the Child suck immediately; if he be an old body let him take it lying in his bed nine days, if it may be conveniently, or otherwise to use no straining.

For a Lask or Flux.

Take one quart of red Wine, as much running water, one ounce of Cinnamon, seeth these half away, and give the patient six spoonfuls to drink morning and evening, if you think it to be too harsh put in a piece of Sugar.

A Lotion Water for the Canker.

Take one gallon of pure Water, four handfuls of Woodbine, of Marigolds, and Tetsul, of each two handfuls, of Celendine, Rue, Sage, and Egrimony, of each one handful, boil all these to a quart, then strain it, and put thereto two great spoonfuls of the best English Honey, and one ounch of Roch-Allum, boil them all again as long as any scum ariseth, then take it off, and put it in a close bottle, and use it blood-warm when need requireth.

For the Mother.

Take three or four handfuls of Ferne that groweth upon a house, seeth it in Renish Wine till it be well sodden, then put it in a linnen cloth, and lay it to her Navel, as hot as she may suffer it, four or five times.

A Water for all old Sores.

Take Honeysuckles, Water Bettany, Rosemary, Sage, Violet leaves, Elder leaves, cut them all small together, and seeth them in a quart of running water, put thereto two spoonfuls of Honey, and a little Allum.

For one that hath a great heat in his Temples, or that cannot sleep.

Take the juyce of Housleek, and of Lettice of each

each one spoonful, of womans Milk six spoonfuls, put them together, and set them upon a Chafing-dish of coals, and put thereto a piece of Rose-cake, and lay it to your Temples.

To quench or slack your thirst.

Take one quart of running water out of the brook, seeth it, and scum it, put thereto five or six spoonfuls of Vinegar, a good quantity of Sugar and Cinnamon, three or four Cloves bruised, drink it luke-warm.

For one that hath a great heat in his hands and stomack.

Take four Eggs, roast them hard, peel them, lay them in Vinegar three or four hours, then let the sick man hold in either hand one of them, and after some space change them and take the other, and it will allay the heat.

Against all Aches especially of a Womans breast.

Take Milk, and Rose-leaves, and set them on the fire, and put thereto Oatmeal, and Oyl of Roses, boil them till they be thick, and lay it hot under the sore, and renew it so till it be always hot.

For the Ptisick and dry Cough.

Take the Lungs of a Fox, beat them to powder, take of Liquorice and Sugar-candy a good quantity, a small quantity of Cummin, mix these all well together, and put them in a bladder; and eat of it as often as you think good in a day.

To take away Warts.

Take Snails that have shells, prick them, and with the juyce that cometh from them, rub the Wart every day for the space of seven or eight days, and it will destroy them.

A perfect water for the sight.

Take Sage, Fennel, Vervin Bettony, Eyebright, Pimpernel, Cinquefoil, and Herb-grace, lay all these in White-wine one night, still it in a stillatory of glass: this Water did restore the sight of one that was blind three years before.

To restore the hearing.

Take Rue, Rosemary, Sage, Vervin, Marjoram, of each one handful, of Cammomil two handfuls, stamp them, and mould them in Rye dough, make thereof one loaf, bake it as other bread, and when it is baked break it in the midst, and as hot as may be suffered bind it to your Ears, and keep them warm and close one day or more, after it be taken away, forbear ye to take cold.

For a Felon in the Joints.

Take Rue, Featherfew, Bores grease, Leaven-Salt, Honey, six leaves of Sage, shred them altogether small, then beat them together, and lay it to the sore place.

To comfort the Brains, and to procure sleep.

Take a red Rose-cake, three spoonfuls of White-wine Vinegar, the white of one Egg, three spoonfuls of womans Milk, set all these on a Chafin-dish of coals, heat them, and lay the Rose-cake upon the dish, and let them heat together, then take one Nutmeg, and strew it on the Cake, then put it betwixt two cloathes, and lay it to your forehead as warm as you may suffer it.

A Medicine for a sore head with a Scald.

Take one peck of Shoo-makers shreds, set them over the fire, in a brass pan, put water to them, and seeth them so long as any Oil will arise, and evermore be scumming off the Oil, then take Plantain, Ribwort, Housleek leaves, Ground Ivy, knotted grass, wild Borrage, Tutsan, Herb-Bennet, Smallage, Setwel leaves, of every one a like quantity, and beat them in a Mortar, and strain them, then take half a Pennyworth of Rosin, half a pennyworth of Allum, a little Virgins Wax, beat them and put them into a pan, and set it over the fire, put thereto the Herbs and the Oil, let them seeth till all be melted, then strain them into a pan, and stir them till they be cold, and put it into a box for your use, when you dress your head, heat a little in a faucer, anoint it every day twice, pull out the hairs that stand upright, and with a linnen cloth wipe away the corruption.

A Salve for a green Wound, or old Sore.

Take the leaves of green Tobacco two pounds, of Valerian two pounds, beat them very small, then strain them, and take the juyce thereof, put one pound of yellow Wax, one pound of Rosin, one pound of Deer Suet, boil them together till they be very green, and when it is cold put to it a quarter of a pound of Turpentine, and keep it for your use

For the running of the Reins, Approved.

Take the Rows of red Herrings, dry them upon the coals till they will beat to pouder, then give it to the patient to drink in the morning fasting, as much as will lye upon a shilling in five spoonfuls of Ale or Wine, be he never so weak.

For the burning and pricking in the Soles of the Feet.

Take half a pound of Barrows greafe, two handfulls of Mugwort chopped very small, boil it with the Barrows greafe upon a soft fire, by the space of four hours, then strain it from the Mugwort, and put it up in an earthen thing for your use, and anoint your feet as you go to bed.

A Medicine for any Heat, Burning or Scalding: Approved.

Take half a pint of the best Cream you can get, and set it in a fair Pofnet, upon the fire, then take 2 good handfuls of Daifie roots, leaves and all, clean wafhed, and very finely fhred, put them into the fame Pofnet, and boil it upon the fire, until it be a clear ointment, then strain it through a cloath, and keep it for your use.

G

To make Aqua compofita *to drink for a Surfeit, or a cold ftomack, and to avoid Flegm, and glut from ftomack.*

Take one handful of Rofemary, one good root of Elecampane, one handful of Hop, half a handful of Thyme, half a handful of Sage, fix good crops of red Mints, and as much of Pennireyal, half a handful of Horehound, fix crops of Marjoram, two ounces of Liquorice well bruifed, and fo much of Annife-feeds, then take three gallons of ftrong Ale, and put all the aforefaid things, Ale, and Herbs, into a brafs pot, then fet them upon the fire, and fet your Limbeck upon it, and ftop it clofe with pafte, that there come no Air out, and fo keep it with a foft fire, as other *Aqua vitæ.*

For an Ach in the Joynts.

Take clarified Butter a quarter of a pound, of Cummin one pound, black Sope a quarter of a pound, one handful of Rue, Sheeps Suet 2 ounces, Bay falt one fpoonful, bray thefe together, then fry them with the gall of an Ox: fpread it on a plaifter, and lay it on as hot as you can, and let it lye feven days.

A Plaifter to lay to the Head for a Rheum which runneth at the Eyes.

Take the powder of Rofe-leaves, Rofe-water, and Bettony-water, of each a like quantity, and a little Vinegar, put your powders into the Water and Vinegar, ftill them and temper them, and make them in a Plaifter, and put to it a little powder of *Terra figillata*

A Water to be ufed with the Plaifter above-faid for the fame purpofe.

Take one quart of new Milk, two pounds of green Fennel, a quarter of a pound of Eye-bright, Put the Herbs and Milk into a Stillatory, caft half an ounce of Camphire thereon, and with this water wafh your eyes and temples.

For the Emerhoids : Approved

Take a piece of twany cloth, burn it in a Frying pan to powder, then beat it in a Mortar as fine as may be, searce it, then lay it on brown paper, and with spittle make it plaister-wise, and lay it to the place, and truss it up with cloths.

To break any Sore.

Take hot bread to the quantity of a farthing loaf, grate it, put thereto Sallade Oil three or four spoonfuls, and a pint of Milk, and seeth them together to a good thickness, spread it on a cloth, and lay it to the sore; instead of Sallade Oil you may use Deer-suet.

A Bath for an Ach in the Back and Limbs.

Take Mugwort, Vervain, Fetherfeu, Dill, Rosemary, Burnet, Tunhoof, Horehound, and white Mints, Senkel, and Sage, of each one handful, seeth all these in four gallons of running-water, and let it seeth till one gallon be wasted, then bath your legs with it five nights together,

A Medicine for any Joynt that is Numb with any Ach. Approved

Take Virgin Wax one ounce, Verdigriece half a quarter of an ounce, Brimstone Sope, oil of eggs, of Allum, of Hony, of each a like quantity, temper them all together, and lay it upon the place grieved somewhat warm.

A Medicine for a Fellon of any Finger.

Take as much Bay-salt as an Egg, wind it in gray paper, lay it in the embers a quarter of an hour, then beat it in a Mortar very fine, then take the yolk of a new laid Egg, beat it with this powder until it be very stiff; spread it upon a cloth, lay it upon the joynt griev'd twenty four hours, and so dress it three times.

For a Boil or Push.

Take the yolk of a new laid Egg, a little English Hony, put it into the shell to the yolk, put in as much Wheat meal as will make it to spread, then take 1 branch of Rue, and 1 branch of Fetherfew, shred them very fine, and put it to the same Medicine, stir them very well together, spread it upon a peace of leather, and lay it to the place grieved.

An Electuary to cause good digestion, and to comfort the stomack.

Take Setwel, and, Gallingal of each three slices, Nutmegs, Ginger, and Cinnamon, of each two slices, three Bay-berries sliced fine and husked, three slices of Liquorice, half a spoonful of Annise-seeds clean dusted, one long Pepper cut small, white Pepper six grains, as much black Pepper, beat them all into a gross pouder, then put thereto two grains of Musk, one grain of Ambergriece, then take Mint-water and Sugar, boil them together and when they are come to the right perfection of thickness, put in those pouders above mentioned in the cooling, with a little Conserve of Rosemary flowers; of this take the quantity of a Nutmeg half an hour before you eat or dring at meals.

A Pouder for the Rheum, or Sore Eyes.

Boil one pint of Hop-water, made when the Hop is in the flower, till it be scalding hot, then put into it half a pound of Liquerice in very fine pouder, the water being taken from the fire, for the Liquorice must not boil in the Water, stir them together till the Water, be clean consumed, then add to them of Annise-seeds, and Fennel-seeds of each half a pound made into very fine pouder through a searce, Angelica-roots, Elicampane roots and leaves, and flowers of Eyebright made into very fine pouder, of each one ounce and a half, mingle these together, and so keep it close, and when you eat of this pouder weigh out of the whole quantity two ounces, whereunto add as much good *Aqua vitæ* as will moisten it or Angelica water, or *Rosa solis*, to keep it from being musty, set it near the fire, eat

of

of this pouder at any time as much as you may take up with a groat, and it is special good for the Rheum, for cold, or for sore eyes. Mr. *Bendlow*.

A Salve for any Wound.

Take Rosin, Per-rosin, Wax, of each eight ounces, of Sheeps Suet, and Frankincense, of each four ounces, one ounce of Mastick made in powder, boil all these in a pint of White-wine half an hour, then take it from the fire, and put thereto half an ounce of Camphire in powder when it is almost cold put thereto four ounces of Turpentine, and make it up in rouls, but before it be rouled you must wash it up in running Water. A. T.

How to deliver a Child in danger.

Take a Date stone, beat it into powder, let the Woman drink it with Wine, then take Polipody and emplaister it to her feet, and the Child will come whether it be quick or dead; then take Centory, green or dry, give it the Woman to drink in wine, give her also the Milk of another Woman.

A most singular Sirrup for the Lungs, and to prevent a Consumption.

Take Egrimony, Scabios, Borrage, Bugloss, of each twenty leaves, Fole-foot, Lungwort, Maidenhair, of each half a handful, Succory and Endive, of each six leaves, of *Carduus benedictus*, Horehound, Nip, of each four crops, unset Hop half a handful, Fennel-roots, Parsly-roots, Smallage-roots, of each three roots sliced and the piths taken out, Elecampane four roots sliced, Iris-roots half an ounce sliced, Quince seeds one ounce, Liquorice three good sticks scraped and sliced small, twenty Figs sliced, Raisins of the Sun one good handful sliced, and the stones taken out, boil all these in a gallon of running water till half be consumed, then take it from the fire and let it settle, then strain it, and boil it again with as much white Sugar as will make it thick as Sirrup, that it may last all the year.

A Choice Manual, or,

A Powder for the Stone.

Take Haws and Hips, of each a good handful, Ashen-keyes half a handful, three or four Acorns, the shells of three new laid Eggs, Grumwel seeds, Parsley-seeds, of each half an ounce, Per-stone a good handful, Camock roots half a handful, make all these in fine powder, then put thereto two ounces of Sugar-candy beaten something small, take a six-penny weight of this powder at a time in the morning fasting, and drink not after it one hour.

For the Chollick and Stone.

Take one handful of *Philipendula*, of Rosemary, of Saxifrage, of Ivy growing on the wall, of Hartstongue, of Thyme, of Parsley, of Scabious, of each four handfuls, of Marigolds one handful, of Marjoram three handfuls, of brown fennel, of Londeheef, of Spernits, of Borrage, of each two handfuls, of Maiden-hair three handfuls, still all these in *May*, keep it in a Glass till you have need of it, then take of it five spoonfuls, and three of White-wine, and of clean powder of Ginger half a spoonful, put these together, and warm it lukewarm, and let the Patient drink it in the morning two hours before he rise out of his bed, let him lay more cloaths upon him, for it will provoke him to sweat, after the sweat is gone, let him rise and walk whither he will.

A good water to drink with wine, or without to cool Choller.

Take Borrage-roots, and Succory-roots of each two, wash and scrape them fair and clean, and take out their cores, then take an earthen pot of two gallons, fill it with fair spring water, set it on a fire of Char-coal, put the roots in it, and eight penny-worth of Cinnamon; when it beginneth to seeth, put into it four ounces of fine Sugar, and let it seeth half an hour, then take it off, let it cool, and drink thereof at your Pleasure.

How to make Aqua composita *for the Chollick and Stone.*

Take strong Ale one Month old, as many gallons as your pot will hold, and for every gallon take two ounces of Liquorice, and as much Annise-seeds, and of these Herbs following two handfuls of each to every gallon, of Beach-leaves, Burnet, Paspher, Pellitory of the wall, Watercresses, Saxafrage, Grumwel, *Philipendula*, Penny-royal, Fennel, half a root of Elecampane, of Hawes, of Hips, of Berries, of Brambles, and Barberries, of each half a pint, still them as you do other *Aqua vitæ*.

A Medicine for the Chollick passion

Take the smooth leaves of Holly, dry them, and make them into powder, of Grumwel-seed, and Box-seed of each a little quantity, let the Patient drink thereof.

How to take away the fervent shaking and burning of an Ague.

Take of the rind of the Wildin-tree, with the leaves in Summer, of each half a handful, as much Bettony, three crops of Rosemary, seeth them in a quart of Posset-Ale to a pint, and let the sick drink of this as hot as he can, and so within three times it will ease him.

For the Hardness or Stiffness of Sinews.

Take twelve fledg'd Swallows out of the nest, kill them, beat them feathers and all in a Mortar, with Thyme, Rosemary, and Hop, then seeth them with May Butter a good while, then strain them through a Strainer, as hard as you can, and it will be an Ointment, take the strings that grow out of the Strawberries, and beat them amongst the rest.

How to stay the Flux.

Take white Starch made of Wheat, two or three spoonfuls, and take also new Milk from the Cow, stir these together, and let them be warmed a little, and

and give it to the Party grieved in manner of a glister; a present Remedy.

An approved Medicine for the Plague called the Philosophers Egg; it is a most excellent preservative, against all Poysons, or dangerous Diseases that draw towards the Heart.

Take a new laid Egg, and break a hole so broad as you may take out the white clean from the Yolk, then take one ounce of Saffron and mingle it with the yolk, but be careful you break not the shell, then cover it with another piece of shell so close as is possible, then take an earthen pot with a close cover, with warm embers, so that he shall not be burned, and as those embers do cool, so put in more hot; and do so for the space of two days untill you think it be dry, for proof whereof you shall put in a Pen, and if it come out dry it is well, then take the Egg and wipe it very clean, then pare the shell, from the Saffron, and set it before the fire, and let it be warm, then beat it in a Mortar very fine, and put it in by it self, then take as much white Mustard-seed as the Egg and Saffron, and grind it as small as meal, then searce it through a fine Boulter, that you may save the quantity of the Egg so searced, then take a quarter of an ounce of Dittany roots, as much Turmentil, of *Nuces Vomicæ* one dram, let them be dryed by the fire as aforesaid, then stamp these three last severally very fine in a Mortar, then mix them three well together, after that, take as a thing most needful, the root of Angelica and Pimpernel, of each the weight of sixpence, make them to powder, and mix them with the rest, then compound therewith five or six scruples of Unicorns-horn, or for want thereof Harts-Horn, and take as much weight as all these fine powders come to, of fine Triacle, and stamp it with the Powders in a Mortar until it be well mixt and hang to the pestle, and then it is perfectly made,

then

then put the Electuary in a stone Pot, well nealed, and so it will continue twenty or thirty years, and the longer the better.

How to use this Electuary.

First, When one is infected with the Pestilence, let him take so soon as he can, or ever the disease infect the heart, one crown weight in gold of this Electuary, and so much of fine Triacle, if it be for a man, but if it shall be for a woman or child take less, and let them be well mixed together, and if the Disease come with cold, give him the Electuary with half a pint of White-wine warm, and well mixed together, but if it come with heat then give it him with Plantain Water, or Well water, and Vinegar mixt together, and when he hath drunk the same, let him go to his naked bed and put off his shirt, and cover him warm, but let his bed be well warmed first, and a hot double sheet wrapped about him, and so let him sweat seven, eight, or ten hours, as he is able to endure, for the more he doth sweat the better, because the disease fadeth away with the sweat, but if he cannot sweat, then heat two or three Bricks or Tiles, and wrap them in moist cloaths wet with Water and Salt, lay them by his sides in the bed, and they will cause him to sweat, and as he sweateth, let it be wiped from his body with dry hot cloths being conveyed into the bed, and his sweat being ended, shift him into a warm bed with a warm shirt, and all fresh new clothes, using him very warily for taking of cold, and let his cloaths that he did sweat in be well aired and washed, for they be infectious; and let the keepers of the sick beware of the breath or Air of the party in the time of his sweating, therefore let her muffle her self with double old cloth, wherein is Wormwood, Rue, Fetherfew, crums of sour Bread and Vinegar, and a little Rose-water, beat all these together, and put it into the Muffler made new

every

every day while you do keep him, and let the sick Party have of it bound in a cloth to smell on while he is in a sweat, then after do it away and take a new, and because he shall be faint and distempered after his Sickness, he shall eat no flesh, nor drink wine the space of nine days, but let him use these Conservatives for his Health, as Conserve of Buglos, Borrage, and red Roses, and especially he shall drink three or four days after he hath sweat, morning and evening, three ounces of the juice of Sorrel, mixed with an ounce of Conserve of Sorrel, and so use to eat and drink whatsoever is comfortable for the Heart, also if one take the quantity of a Pea of the said Electuary with some good Wine, it shall keep him from the Infection, therefore when one is sick in the house of the Plague, then so soon as you can, give all the whole Houshold some of this Receipt to drink, and his Keeper also, and it shall preserve them from the Infection, yet keep the whole from the sick as much as you can, beware of the cloaths and bed that the sick Party did sweat in.

To make Balm water.

Take four gallons of strong Ale and stale, half a pound of Liquorice, two pound of Balm, two ounces of Figs, half a pound of Annise-seeds, one ounce of Nutmegs, shred the Balm and Figs very small, and let them stand steeping four and twenty hours, and then put it in a Still as you use *Aqua vitæ.*

To make Doctor Stevens Water.

Take one gallon of good Gascoin Wine, of Ginger, Galingal, Nutmegs, Grains, Annise-seeds, Fennel seeds, Carraway seeds, Sage, Mints, red Roses, garden Thyme, Pellitory, Rosemary, wild Thyme, Penny-royal, Cammomil, Lavender, of each one handful, bray your Spices small, and chop the Herbs before named, and put them with the Spices

spices into the Wine, and let it stand twelve hours, stirring it very often, then still it in a Limbeck, closed up with course paste, so that no Air enter, keep the first water by it self, it is good so long as it will burn.

An Ointment for any strain in the Joynts, or for any Sore.

Take three pounds of fresh Butter unwashed, and set it in an Oven after the bread be drawn out, and let it stand two or three hours, then take the clearest of the butter, and put into a Posner, then take the Tops of red Nettles as much as will be moistned with the Butter, and chop them very small, and put them into the Butter, set it on the fire, and boil it softly 5 or 6 hours, and when it is so boiled put thereto half a pint of pure oyl Olive, and then boil it a very little, and take it off, and strain it into an earthen pot, and keep it for your use.

If you think good, instead of Nettles only, you may take these herbs, Cammomil, Rosemary, Lavender, Tun-hoof, otherwise Ale-hoof, Five-finger, Vervain, and Nettle-tops.

For an Ague.

Take the inner bark of a Walnut-tree, a good quantity, boil it in Beer until the Beer look black, and then take a good draught and put it into a pot, then take six spoonfuls of Sallade Oil, for an extream Ague, brew it to and fro in two pots, then drink it, and let the party labour at any exercise until he sweat, then let him lye down upon a bed very warm until he hath done sweating, this do three times when the Ague cometh upon him.

A Powder against the wind in the Stomack.

Take Ginger, Cinnamon, and Galingal, of each two ounces, Annise-seeds, Catraway, and Fennel-seeds, of each one ounce, long Pepper, Grains, Mace, and Nutmegs, of each half an ounce, Setwel half a drachm, make all in powder, and put thereto one pound of white Sugar, and use this after your Meat, or before at your pleasure, at all times;

it comforteth the stomack marvellously, carrieth away the wind, and causeth a good digestion.

For a Pin and Web in the Eye.

Take the white of an Egg, beat it to oyl, put thereto a quarter of a spoonful of English Hony, half a handful of Daisie leaves, and in winter the roots, half a handful of the inner rind of a young Hazle, not above one years growth, beat them together in a Mortar, and put thereto one spoonful of Womans Milk, and let it stand infused, two or three hours, and strain all through a cloth, and with a feather drop it into the eye thrice a day.

For blood shotten and sore Eyes, coming of heat.

Take *Tutty*, of *Alexandria*, or *Lapis Tutty*, one ounce, beat it unto fine pouder, temper it with a quart of White wine put thereto one ounce of dried Rose-leaves, and boil them altogether with a soft fire until one half be consumed, then strain it through a fine linnen cloth and keep it in a Glass, and use it evening and morning, and put it into the sore eyes with a feather, or your finger.

If the *Tutty* be prepared it is the better, which is thus done, steep the *Tutty* in Rose-water, and let it lye half an hour, then take it forth, and lay it on a white paper to dry, then take it when it is dry, steep it, and dry it again, as before, twice or thrice, and then use it as before,

For an Ach in the Bones.

Take Southernwood, Wormwood, and Bay-leaves, of each one handful, one Oxe-gall, one pint of Neats-foot oil, put all these together, and let them stand two or three days, and let them boil upon a very soft fire, then put in of Deers-suet a good quantity, strain them, and put them into a pot, and so anoint the Patient, put to this a good quantity of Tar, and as much Pitch as the bigness of of a Walnut, and of the juyce of Pimpernel a good quantity.

For Children that are troubled with an extream Cough.

Take Hyſop-water, and Fennel-water, of each half a pint, of ſliced Liquorice, and Sugar, of each a pretty quantity, ſeeth them eaſily over a good fire; ſtrain it, and let them take a little hereof at once, and often; you may diſſolve pellets therein, and you may anoint their cheſt with oyl of Almonds, and a little Wax.

A Medicine for ſore Eyes.

Take red Fennel and Celendine, of each one handful, ſtamp and ſtrain them, that done, take five ſpoonfuls of Honey, and white Copperas the quantity of one Pea, Roſe-water five ſpoonfuls, boil all theſe together in an earthen pot, skim it well, and clarifie it with the white of an Egg; this is an excellent Medicine to clear the ſight of the Eye, if there be any thing in the Eye ſuperfluous to hinder the ſight, but if their be nothing but heat, it is nothing ſo good.

To help one that is inwardly bruiſed.

Take of Borrage and red Sage of each a handful, ſtamp theſe together, and ſtrain them, and put thereto as much Claret Wine as the juyce thereof, and let the Party drink it warm, and if it keep within him four and twenty hours after he will recover; if he be bound in the Body, let him take three ſpoonfuls of Sirrup of Damask Roſes, and two ſpoonfuls of Sallade Oil, and drink it Faſting, and an hour after let the Party take ſome Warm Broth.

For the Spleen.

Take of Lavender, Fennel, Parſley, Cammomile, Thyme, Wormwood, Angellica, of each one handful, of Sage, and Rue, one handful, of Anniſe-ſeeds, and Fennel-ſeeds, of each one handful, of Cummin-ſeeds two handfuls, of Cloves four ſpoonfuls,

fuls, and of Mace two spoonfuls, gather these Herbs in the heat of the Day, and dry them in the Sun two days, laying them very thin on a sheet, and bruise the seed grosly, and steep them in as much Sallade oile as will cover all these things, and somewhat more, and set them in the Sun ten days, which being done, strain your Oyl from your Herbs and your Spices, and then infuse it once again as before with Herbs and Spices in like manner, and to that Oyl thus infused or strained, add bitter Almonds, and Oyl of Capers half a pint, then then take a quarter of a spoonful of the said Oyl, and put it in your hands, your hands being warm, rub them together, and anoint and rub the patient grieved with both your hands, the one on the right side, the other on the left, from the loyns down to the bottom of the belly, drawing your hands as hard as you can, and make them to meet at the bottom of the belly: And continue in continual rubbing about a quarter of an hour.

For a Burning or Scald

Take a quantity of sheeps Suet, the white of Hen-dung, and fresh grease, boil all these together, strain it and anoint the party with a feather.

For the Emerhoids and Piles.

Take juyce of Elder, May-butter, and Deers-suet, melt them, letting the juyce and the butter simmer, and then put the Suet to them, make them in pills, and if you make a suppositor, you must put in more Deers-suet.

For the Canker in the Mouth or Nose.

Take the ashes of green leaves of Holly, with half so much of the burnt powder of Allum, blow with a Quill into the place grieved, and it will help Man, Child, or Beast.

A Remedy for the Mother.

When the Fit beginneth to take them, take the powder of white Amber, and burn it in a Chafing-dish

dish of coals, and let them hold their Mouths over it, and suck in the smoak, and anoint their Nostrils with the oyl of Amber, and if they be not with Child, take two or three drops of the oyl of Amber in White-wine warm or cold, but the oyl of Amber must be taken inward but once a day, and outward as often as the Fit taketh them.

A Medicine for the Worms.

Take one penny-worth of Aloes, with the like quantity of Ox-gall and Mithridate, mix them together, and lay them to the Childs navel upon a Plaister.

A Preservative against the Plague.

Take one dry Walnut, take off the shell and peel, cut it small, and with a branch of Rue shred fine, and a little Wine Vinegar and Salt, put all into a sliced Fig, take it up fasting, and then you may drink a little Wormwood after it, and go where you list.

A Pill for those that are infected.

Take of Aloes-Succatrina half an ounce, of Myrrh, and English Saffron, of each a quarter of an ounce, beat them into small powder, with Malmsey, or a little Sack, or Dioscoridon, make two or three small pills thereof, and take them fasting.

A Poultess to break a Plague-Sore.

Take a white Lilly root, and seeth it in a penny-worth of Linseed, and a pretty quantity of Barrows grease, beat the Linseed first very soft, afterwards beat all together in a Mortar, make thereof a plaister.

An Electuary for the Plague.

Take the weight of ten grains of Saffron, two ounces of the kernels, of Walnuts, two or three Figs, one dram of Mithridate, and a few Sage leaves stampt together, with a sufficient quantity of Pimpernel-water, make up all these together in a Mass or lump, and keep it in a glass or pot for your use, take the quantity of twelve grains fasting in the morning, and it will not only preserve from the Pestilence, but expel from those that are infected.

Against a Tertian Ague.

Take *Dandilion* clean washed, stamp it and put it in Beer, and let it stand all night in the Beer, in the morning strain it, and put half a spoonful of Triacle into it, make it luke-warm, and let the patient drink of it fasting upon his well day, and walk upon it as long as he is able, this hath been approved good for an Ague that cometh every second day.

Against the Wind.

Take Cummin-seeds, and steep them in Sack four and twenty hours, dry them by the fire, and hull them, then take Fennel-seed, Carraway-seed, and Annise-seeds, beat all these together, and take every morning half a spoonful in Broth or Beer fasting.

Another.

Take Enula Campana, grate it, and drink half a spoonful fasting.

For the Sting of an Adder.

Take a head of Garlick, and bruise it with some Rue, and some Hony thereto, and if you will some Triacle, and apply it to the place.

For the biting of a dog.

Take Ragwort, chop it, and boil it with unwasht butter to an ointment.

A Medicine for a Woman that hath a dead Child, or for the after-birth after Deliverance.

Take Date-stones, dry them and beat them to powder, then take Cummin seed, Grains and English Saffron, make them in a powder, and put them altogether in like quantity, saving less of the Saffron then of the rest, then searce them very finely, and when need is to drink it, take a spoonful at once with a little Malmsie, and drink it Milk-warm, it is good to bring forth a dead Child, or for the after-

after-birth, or if the woman have any rising in her stomach, or flushing in her face during her Childbirth the Date stones with round holes in the sides are the best; if you put a quantity of white Amber beaten amongst the powder, it will be better.

To make the best Paracelsus *Salve.*

Take of Litharge of Gold and Silver, of each three ounces, and put to it one pound and half of good Sallade oyl, and as much of Linseed oyl, put it into a large earthen Vessel well leaded, of the fashion of a Milk-boul, or a great Bason, set it over a gentle fire, and keep it stirring till it begin to boil, then put to it of red lead, and of *Lapis Calaminaris*, of each half a pound, keep it with continual stirring, and let it boil two hours, or so long till it be something thick, which you may know by dropping a little of it upon a cold board or stone, then take a Skillet, and put into it a pound of yellow Wax, as much black Rosin, half a pound of Gum Sandrach, of yellow Amber, Olibanum, Myrrh, of *Aloes hepatica*, of both the kinds of *Aristolochias* round and long, of every of these in fine powder searced one ounce, of *Mammir* one ounce and a half, of oyl of Bayes half a pound, of oyl of Juniper six ounces, dissolve all these together in the aforesaid Skillet, and then put them to the former Plaister, set it over a gentle fire; and keep it with stirring till it boil a little. Then take your five Gums, Pepanax, Galbanum, Sapagenum, Ammoniacum, and Bdelium, of each of these three ounces, which must be dissolved in White-wine Vinegar, and strained, and the Vinegar exasperated from them, before you go about the Plaister; let there be three ounces of each of them when they are thus prepared, then when the Plaister hath gently boiled, about half the bigness of a Nutmeg at a time, continuing that order until all the Gums be in and dissolved, then set it over the fire again, and let it boil a very little, but before it boil be sure that the Gums be all dissolved, for else it will run into lumps and knots, after it hath boiled a little take it from the fire again, and continue the stirring of it very carefully, and put to it these things following, being in a readiness, take of both the Corrals red and white, of Mother of Pearl, Dragons blood, *Terra lemnia*, of white Vitriol, of each of them one ounce, of *Lapis hematitis*, and of the Loadstone, of each of them one ounce and a half, of the flowers of Antimony two drams, of *Crocus Martis* two drams, of Camphire one ounce, and of common Turpentine half a pound, mix all these together, but first let those things that are to be pounded, be carefully done, and fully searced, then put them all together among the former things, and again set it over the fire with a moderate heat, and gentle to boil, till it be in the form of a Plaister, which you may know by dropping it on a cold piece of Wood, or Stone, or Iron, you must also remember to keep it with continual stirring, from the beginning to the ending, when you make it up, let your hands, and the place you roul it on, be anointed with the oil of Sain-Johns wort, and of each Worms and Juniper, Cammomil and Roses together, wrap it in Parchment or Leather, and keep it for your use.

Memorandum, That the Camphire be dissolved in the Oyl of Juniper, mix them together with the Gum Sandrach, and put them in towards the latter end.

An Ointment for any strain in the Joynts, or for any Sore.

Take three pound of fresh Butter unwashed, and and set it into an Oven after the bread be drawn out, and let it stand 2 or 3 hours, then take the clearest of the Butter, and put into a posnet, then take the tops of red Nettles, and chop them very small, and

and put so many Nettles to the Butter, as will be moistned with the Butter, and so set it on the fire, and boil it softly five or six hours, and when it is so boiled, put thereto half a pint of the best Oil Olive, and then make it boil a very little, and take it off, and strain it into an earthen pot, and keep it for your use.

Mr Ashleys *Ointment*.

Take six pound of *May* Butter unsalted, one quart of Sallade Oil, four pound of Barrows grease, one pound of the best Rosin, one pound of Turpentine, half a pound of Frankincense: To this rate take these herbs following, of each a handful, viz. Smallage, Balm, Lorage, red Sage, Lavender, Lavender-cotten, Herb-grease, Parsley, Cumfry called Boneset, Sorel, Laurel-leaves, Beach-leaves, Lungwort, Marjoram, Rosemary, Mallows, Cammomile, Saint-*Johns*-wort, Plantain Al'heal, Chickweed, English Tobacco, or else Henbane, Grumsel, Woundwort, Bettony, Agrimony, *Carduus Benedictus*, wild Wine, or White-wine, called Brian, Adders tongue, Mellilot, pick all these herbs clean, wash them, strain them clean from the water, all these must be gathered after the Sun rise, then stamp all these Herbs in a stone or wooden Mortar so small as possible may be, then take your Rosin and beat it to powder with your Frankincense, and melt them first alone, then put in your Butter, your Hogs-grease and Oyl, and when all is melted, put in your Herbs, and let them all boil together half a quarter of an hour, then take it from the fire, and leave stirring of it in no wise a quarter of an hour after, and in that time that it is from the fire put in your Turpentine, and two ounces of Verdigriece very finely beaten to powder, and when you put in your Turpentine and Verdigriece, stir it well, or else it will run over, and so stir until it leave boiling: Then put it in an earthen pot, stopping

the

the pot very close with a cloth, and a board on the top, and set it in a dunghil of Horse muck twenty one days, then take it up and put it into a kettle, and let it boil a little, taking heed that it boil not over, then strain all through a course cloth into an earthen or gally-pot, and when all is strained, put to it half a pound of oyl of Spike, and cover the pot close until you use it, and when you use it make it warm in Winter, and use it cold in Summer.

An approved Medicine for any Ach in the Joynts whatsoever.

Take half a pound of Rosin, half a pound of Frankincense, Olibanum, and Mastick, of each one ounce, Wax, Deers-suet, Turpentine, of each two ounces, Camphire, two drams, beat the Olibanum, Mastick, Rosin, and Frankincense, and Camphire into Powder, then put it in a brass pan with a Pottle of White-wine, and put in the Wax, and Deerssuet into it, and when it doth boil put in your Turpentine, and let it boil a quarter of an hour, then take it from the fire and let it stand and cool until the next day, then work it with your hand to work out the Wine, anointing your hands first with oyl, then make it up in rouls, then as need shall serve, take thereof and spread it with a warm knife upon a fleshy side of a Sheeps-skin, and apply it warm to the grieved place, and take it not off until it fall off of it self, pricking the Plaister full of holes.

A Searcloth to be used against Carbuncles, red Sores, Biles, Swellings, or any hot cause.

Take a wine pint of pure Sallade oyl, and put it into an earthen pot that is very large, and set it upon a very soft fire of Charcoal, and when it beginneth to boil, stir it with a Hasel-stick of one years shooting, then put into it two ounces of *Venice* Sope that is pure white, half a pound of red Lead,

Lead, one quarter of a pound of white Lead, letting it boil very softly, stirring it continually with this Hazle stick for the space of two or three hours; you shall know when it is boiled by this, drop one drop thereof on a board, and it will be stiff when it is enough, then take it from the fire, and put into it half an ounce of oyl of Bays, then let it boil again a little, then let your cloaths be cut of a reasonable size to dip them in it, then you must have two sticks, which must be hollow in the middle to strip the cloaths through, then lay them abroad until they be cold upon a board, then roul them up and keep them, and when you use them, lay them upon the place grieved, and let them lye twelve hours, then take it off and wipe it, and lay the other side, and let that lye as long.

Plague water to be taken three times, for the first helpeth not.

Take a gallon of White-wine, Ale or Beer, and to that quantity take a quarter of a pound of each of these Herbs following, Rosewater a quarter of a pint, Rue, Sage, Vervin, Egrimony, Bettony, Celendine, Carduus, Angelica, Pimpernel, Scabious, Valerian, Worm-wood, Dragons, Mugwort, all these Herbs must you shred in gross together, and steep it in the aforesaid liquor, the night before you distil it in a Rose-water Still, and then keep the first water by it self, being the weaker, and therefore fitter for Children; it helpeth all Fevers, Agues and Plagues being thus taken, seven spoonfuls or thereabout of the strongest blood-warm, and give to the party to drink in an Ague or Fever, an hour before the Fit come, and so to sweat, either by Exercise, or in your bed, but your Stomach must be empty, if it be taken for the Plague, then put it into a little Diascordium or Mithridate.

A defensive Plaister.

Take the White of an Egg, and Bole Armoniack, spread it on leather.

A Sirrup for a Cold.

Take Colts-foot-water, Hysop-water, and Hony, put Liquorice, Annise-seeds, Elecampane, put thereto the juyce of Fennel, and boil them.

To stay the bleeding of a Wound.

Take Charcoal, red hot out of the fire and beat it to Powder.

A Poultess.

Take Milk, Oatmeal, and red Rose-leaves, and a little Deers-suet.

For the running of the Reins.

Take Cups of Acorns and grate them, and grate some Nutmeg, put this in Beer and drink.

For a Poultess.

Take Linseed and beat it to pouder, boil it in Milk with Mallows, and Sheeps-suet.

For a Blast

Taste a good quantity of Vervin, and boil it in Milk, and wash the blast therewith very well, then bind the Herbs very close to it some few hours, after wash it again the Milk being warmed, and so bind it up again, the oftner it is done the better, and in a day or two it will be well, if it be taken before it fester.

Another.

Take a good quantity of Vericon being green, with as much Dill, chop them together, and boil them in Bores grease as much as will cover them, and for want thereof so much *May* butter, and when they be boiled together, let them stand two or three days, and then boil it a little, and so strain it through a cloth.

A Balsamum.

Take it in the latter end of *September*, good store of Honysuckle-berries and put them in a body of a glass still stopped, and set it in hot horse-dung eight days, distil it in Balneo, then when you have drawn the water forth, pour the water into the
stuff

stuff again, stop it close, and put it into the dung four and twenty hours, then set it in ashes, and distil both Water and Oyl with a great fire, as much as will come forth, and at last separate the water from the Oyl in Balneo.

To make an excellent Oil of Hypericon.

Take flowers, leaves and seeds of Hypericon, as much as you list, beat them together, and infuse them in White-wine, that they may be covered therewith, and set them in the Sun for ten days, then put thereto so much Oyl Olive as all the rest do weigh, and let it stand ten days more in the Sun, but look that you weigh the Oyl to know how much it is, then put thereto for every pound of Oyl two ounces of Turpentine, and one dram of Saffron, and of Nutmegs, and Cloves of each half an ounce, of Myrrh, and Rosin, of each an ounce, and of the Root of Briony two ounces put them all in a vessel of glass, and mix them well together, and set them in a vessel of hot water, and then set thereto a head of glass and Receiver well shut, and boil it so long until no more will distil from it, which will be about twenty four hours, then take it out and strain it whilst it is hot, and keep it in a vessel of glass, and when you first use it, heat it well, and apply it upon a wound without using any tent at all, this is excellent for a green wound, especially if there be veins, sinews, or bones offenced or cut, it keepeth wounds from putrifaction, it cleanseth them, and easeth pain, and doth incarnate and skin them, it helpeth bruises, pains, aches, or swelling in any part, and is wonderful good against venome or poyson.

For the Falling-sickness.

Take the roots of single Pionies grate them, drink them, and wear some of them about your neck.

For the kibed Heels.

Take a Turnip, make a hole in the top of it, take

take out some of the pith, infuse into that hole Oyl of Roses, then stop close the hole, roast the Turnip under the embers, when it is soft, apply it plaister-wise warm to the Kibe, bind it fast.

Lapis Prunellæ.
A Medicine for sore Eyes.

Take one pound of Salt-peter, boil it in a Goldsmiths earthen pot, with a very hot fire round about it, let it boil till it be very black and melted, then take a quarter of an ounce, or sixpeny weight of Roach Allum, and a quarter of an ounce of Brimstone, break them and put them in the Salt-peter by little at once as it boileth, and let it burn till the flame go out of it self, then pour it into a brass Ladle, or into a Chafer, and so let it stand till it be cold, and when you will use it scrape it very fine with a knife, and put a little of it to the sore eyes, hold down the eye-lid till the pain be gone, then let the water drop out of the eye: This Medicine taketh away the Pearl, Pin and Web in the eye, and all sores and blood shed, it also helpeth the tooth-ach, being put into the hollow tooth, with a little lint, if the tooth be not hollow, rub it outward; finally, it helpeth a stinking breath, being eaten in the morning fasting.

For a Scald Head.

Take a handful of Glovers shreds, and a handful of Dock-roots the pith taken out, and boil them in strong Ale until they be reasonable thick, and anoint the head therewith.

For a Bloody-Flux.

Take Rubarb and toast it, then grind it to powder, and take as much as will lye upon a sixpence, and keep warm that day, the next day eat conserve of Roses, mixed with Corral, and drink that day if you will posset-Ale made of Cammomil.

For the Itch.

Take a pound of Butter, unwashed and unsalted, three

three good handfuls of red Sage, and as much Brimstone beaten into powder, as a Walnut, boil these well together, and strain it, and put in half an ounce of Ginger beaten small.

For sore eyes.

Take two Hens dung out of the nest, and put it into an Oven almost cold, let it lye there all night, and take the white of it, and beat it being dryed, and take as much of the powder of Ginger finely beaten, and put to that half the like quantity of Sugar-candy, all which must be beaten very well and searced, then put it into the sore eyes every night, and in the morning, and wash it out with water.

A water for sore Eyes.

Take a pint of fair running water, of wild Daisies, and three leaved grass, of each a good handful, wash the herbs very clean in a Cullender, and put them into a clean skillet of water, let them boil very well over the fire, until the water look green, then take a little piece of Allum and put into the water, and when it is boiling then tast of the water, and when it sticks to the mouth, take as much honey as will make it very sweet, then after it hath boiled a little while, take it off the fire, strain it, and drop a little every night into the eyes.

An approved Application against any Surfeit.

Take the bottom of a Muncorn loaf, cut it about an inch thick, and as broad as the palm of your hand, toast it very well, then take of Sallade oil and Claret wine of each a like quantity, as much as will wet the toast well and throughly, warm it hot, then put the toast into it, when the toast is well soak'd, strew the powder of Cloves, and Mace hereupon thick, then apply it to the stomach of the patient as warm as he can endure it, it will purge upwards and downwards, so often as you apply a fresh toast made as aforesaid

said, that may be applyed so often as any one findeth their stomach ill at ease, although then it will not purge, except in case of a surfeit.

A Medicine against the Plague.

Take of the root called Setwel, the quantity of half a Walnut, and grate it, of Triacle green one good spoonful, of fair water three spoonfuls, make all these more than luke-warm, and so drink them off in bed, and sweat six or seven hours, and in your sweat drink small Posset-ale, made of small drink as you need, but not till an hour and half after the taking of the potion, and it will bring forth the plague, for if you cast the medicine, you may take it the second, third, or fourth time, by the whole, half, or less measure, as your stomach will bear it: if any do take it, and thereupon happen presently amendment, or a rising or sore, you may think it to be the sickness, for the nature of the medicine is to prevent the plague, and in others to expel the sore, if it be not taken too late, in which case the stomach will not brook it easily, and after two or three times taking, if you minister it to any, let it be at their first sickness, lest if their disease be other, they may receive harm thereby.

Jelly of Frogs.

Take the Jelly of Frogs in March, and still it in a glass Still, it is a good Medicine to stop blood, and for the heat and redness of the face, and good to cure green wounds.

For the Tooth-ach.

Take Sparemints, and Ground-ivy, of each a handful, and a good spoonful of Bay Salt, stamp all these very well together, and boil them in a pint of the strongest Vinegar that you can get, let these boil all together until they come to a quarter of a pint, then strain it, and put it into a glass, and stop it very close, when your teeth do ach, Take a
spoon-

spoonful of it blood-warm, and hold it in your mouth on that side the pain is.

To make teeth stand fast.

Take Roots of Vervin in cold wine, and wash the teeth therewith.

For the perilous Cough.

Take white Horehound, stamp it, wring out the juice, and mingle it with honey, and seeth it, and give it to the sick to drink, or else Sack, and Garlick-seed and roast it in the fire. and take away the peeling, and eat the rest with Honey, or else take Sage, Rue, Cummin, and powder of Pepper, and seeth all these together in honey, and make thereof an Electuary, and take thereof a spoonful in the morning, and another at night.

For a man that hath no taste in meat or drink.

Take a pottle of clear water, and a good handful of Dandilion, and put it in an earthen pot, and seeth it till it come to a quart, and then take out the Herbs, and put in a good quantity of white Sugar, till you think it be somewhat pleasant, and then put it into a Vessel wherein it may cool, and then take twenty or thirty Almonds, blanch them and beat them in a mortar, and when the water is cold put it to the Almonds, and strain it through a clean Cipris-bag without compulsion, and if it be thick, let it run through again, and so keep it in a vessel, and drink of it often, at all times as you please.

To preserve a man from the Plague.

Take *Aloe Epaticum*, and *Aloe Succatrina*, fine Cinnamon and Myrrh, of each of them three drams, Cloves, Mace, *Lignum Aloe*, Mastick, *Bole Armoniack*, of each of them half a dram, let all these things be well stamped in a Mortar, then mingle them together, and after keep them in some close vessel, and take of it every morning two penny-weight, in half a glass full of White-wine,

with

with a little water, and drink it in the morning at the dawning of the day, and so may you by the grace of God, go safely into all infection of the air and plague.

For a Tetter or Ring-worm.

Take Mercury a quarter of an ounce, Camphire one penny weight, make them into powder, and rub them in a fair Porrenger, then take and mix them with the water of the Vine four or five spoonfuls, stir them well together, then put as much more water to that, then strain it through a cloth, and take Poppy-seeds one quarter of an ounce, beat that in a stone Mortar with a spoonful of the water of the Vine, putting a little and a little till you have spent the quantity of a pint, then put to half an ounce of the milk of Cokernut, so mix them well together with your Receipt, and strain them as you make Almond milk through a fair cloth, then keep it in a glass for your use.

To keep ones body loose whensoever you need.

Take two ounces of Sirrup of Roses, one ounce of Sene, one penny-worth of Annise-seeds, one stick of Liquorice, one pint of Posturn-water, seeth them all together till it seeth to half a pint, then strain them forth, then boil the two ounces of Sirrup of Roses, and drink it warm.

For a red Face.

Take Brimstone that is whole, and Cinnamon of either of them an even proportion by weight, beat them into small powder, searce it through a fine cloth upon a sheet of white paper, to the quantity of an ounce or more, and so by even proportions in weight, mingle them together in clean clarified Capons-grease, and temper them well together, until they be well mollified, and then put them in a little Camphire to the quantity of a Bean, and so put the whole confection in a glass.

For a young Child to make Water.

Boil Organy in fair Water, and lay it warm to the Childs Navel.

A Medicine for the falling of the Uvula into the Throat.

Take a red Colewort leaf, whereof cut away the middle rind, then put the Leaf into a paper, and let it be burnt in hot embers or ashes, then take the leaf out, and lay it hot on the top or crown of the bare head, and it will draw it up into his place and rid you of your pain.

A Medicine for the heat of the soles of the feet, that cometh by Rheum or Blood

Take a quantity of Snails of the garden, and boil them in stale Urine, then let the patient bath and set his feet therein, and using that often he shall be cured.

Gascoins own Powder.

Take of powder of Pearl, of red Corral, of Crabs-eyes, of Hartshorn, and white Amber, of each one ounce, beat them into fine powder, and searce them, then take so much of the black toes of the Crabs claws as of all the rest of the powders, for that is the chief worker, beat them, and searce them finely as you do the rest, then weigh them severally, and take as much of the toes as you do of all the rest of the five powders, and mingle them well together, and make them up in balls with jelly of Hartshorn, whereinto put or infuse a small quantity of Saffron to give them colour, then let them lie till they be dry and fully hard, and keep them for your use.

The Crabs are to be gotten in *May* or *September*, before they be boiled.

The dose is ten or twelve grains in Dragon water, Carduus water, or some other Cordial water.

The Apothecaries in their composition of it, use to put in a drachm of good Oriental Bezar to the other powders, as you may see in the prescription following.

This is thought to be the true composition invented by *Gascon*, and that the Bezar, Musk, and Ambergriece, were added after by some for curiosity, and that the former will work without them as effectually as with them.

The Apothecaries Gascon powder, *with the use.*

Take of Pearls, white Amber, Harts-horn, eyes of Crabs, and white Corral, of each half an ounce, of black thighs of Crabs calcined, two ounces, to every ounce of this powder put a dram of Oriental Bezar, reduce them all into very fine powder, and searce them, and with Harts-horn jelly, with a little Saffron put therein, make it up into past, and make therewith Lozenges, or Trochises for your use.

You must get your Crabs for this powder about *May* or in *September*, before they shall be boyled, when you have made them, let them dry and grow hard in a dry air, neither by Fire nor Sun.

Their dose is ten or twelve grains, as before prescribed in the former page.

The powder prescribed by the Doctors in their last London Dispensatory 1650 called the powder of Crabs claws.

Take of prepared Pearls, eyes or stones of Crabs, of red Corral, of white Amber, of Hearts-horn, of Oriental Bezar-stone of each half an ounce, of the powder of the black tops of the Crabs-Claws to the weight of all the former; make them all into powder, according to Art, and with jelly made with the skins or castings of our Vipers, make it up into small Tablets, or Trochises, which you must warily dry, as before prescribed, and reserve for your use.

The

The Countess of Kents *powder, good against all malignant and pestilent Diseases;* French Pox, Small Pox, Measels, Plague, Pestilence, *malignant, or scarlet Fevers; good against Melancholy, dejection of Spirits; twenty or thirty grains hereof being exhibited in a little wharm Sack, or Hearts-horn jelly, to a man, and half as much, or twelve grains to a child.*

Take of the Magistery of Pearls, of Crabs-eyes prepared, of white Amber prepared, Hearts-horn, Magistery of white Corral, of *Lapis contra Yarvam*, of each a like quantity, to these powders infused put of the black tips of the great claws of Crabs, the full weight of the rest, beat these all into very fine powder, and fearce them through a fine Lawne Searce, to every ounce of this powder, add a drachm of true Oriental Bezar, make all these up into a lump, or masse, with the jelly of Harts-horn, and colour it with Saffron, putting thereto a scruple of Ambergriece and a little musk also finely powdered, and dry them (made up into small Trochifes) neither by fire nor Sun, but by a dry air; and you may give to a Man twenty grains of it, and to a Child twelve grains.

The vertues of a Root called Contra yerva, *being made into fine Powder.*

1. It withstands the plague being taken in Triacle-water.

2. It is good in all pestilent Diseases, taken in posset drink with Saffron.

3. It is good against a Fever, taken in *Carduus* Water.

4. It is a great Antidote against all Poysons, taken in Sallade Oyl.

5. It doth cure the biting of a mad Dog, drunk in Rose Vinegar, and then drink nothing else but Spring water during the Cure.

6. It causeth a speedy delivery, given in Balm water, Bittony water, or in burnt Wine.

7. It

7. It doth take away the afterthrows, given in the same liquors

8. It is a good Cordial in all fits of the Mother, given in Rue-water.

9. It is very soveraign in swouning Fits given in Sack, or Botrage-water.

10. It is very powerful to withstand all Melancholly, given in Sack.

11. It doth help Convulsions in Children given in Spring-water.

12. It helpeth the Worms given in Goats Milk.

13. It is good for a short Breath, given in Rue-water.

14. It helpeth the Head pain, given in Rue-water, or Rosemary-water.

15. It helpeth the yellow Jaundice, given in Celendine-water.

16. It is very powerful in the Palsie, given in Sage-water.

17. It is a good Antidote against the Gout, given in Sage-water.

18. It withstandeth the growing of the Stone in the Reins, given in Renish-wine.

19. It causeth a good and quiet sleep taken in White-wine.

20. It is a great Preserver of Health, and means of long Life, taken sometimes in Mead.

21. It may be used as Triacle, or Bezar against Surfeits.

22. It is a general upon all Occasions, and may be given at all times, when you do not know what the Disease is, in any of the aforesaid liquors.

The Dose for a Man or Woman, is from one scruple, to two scruples, and a Boy or Girl twelve or fourteen grains, in convenient Liquors.

THE

The EPISTLE.

Friend,

BEing given to understand, that you were reprinting the Countess of Kents Manual; I thought good to communicate unto you, for the more Accomplishment of your second Impression, the Vertues of some select Cordial Spirits, of very great Use in weak and sickly Persons, which were first composed by Sir Walter Raleigh, during his Imprisonment in the Tower, and dispersed by him to divers worthy Personages, in their several Occasions and Necessities, and were imparted to me, by Captain Samuel King, who lived long time with him in the Tower, and in his Expeditions; this King being my loving Friend, and Schoolfellow, both in Canterbury and Westminster Schools; I have also inserted hereunto certain Experiments of Gascons Powder, or the Countesses, for their Operations are much of the same nature, which have many times with very happy Success been tried, upon several Persons by my self, and divers others by my Directions, assuring my self, it will be of very great Use and Benefit to such Persons as shall have need of such Helps and Comforts; and so rest,

Your Friend,
W. J.

The Vertues of Aqua Bezoar.

IT is good against contagious Diseases, as Plague, Purples, spotted Fevers, Small-pox, and Measels.

The Order to take it, is with *Carduus Benedictus*, or Angelica in Posset Ale, and so sweat moderately upon the taking of it; it is good against Surfeits, and easeth the Stomack opprest with Wind, crude flegm, and Superfluities, and helpeth Digestion.

The Dose is from two to three Spoonfuls at one time.

The

The Vertues of Spirit of Clary.

It is good to restore one in any Weakness, chiefly of the back: It preserveth against the Consumption and Ptisick; It comforteth the Heart, and increaseth radical moisture; It also strengtheneth Child bearing Women after their Delivery.

The Dose is one or two Spoonfuls morning and evening.

The Vertues of Aqua Mariæ.

It is good for all Infirmities of the Spleen, and to open the Obstructions thereof, it comforteth the vital parts, and is good against all Passions of the Heart; it preserveth the Meat in the Stomack from Putrifaction; it helpeth Digestion, and expelleth Wind.

The Dose is one spoonful at one time.

The Vertues of Flowers of Rosemary.

It is good against all Infirmities of the Stomack, and to suppress all offensive fumes rising up from thence to the head, keeping them down, and helpeth Memory; It openeth all stoppings of the Liver and Melt, it preventeth *Vertigo, Scotomia,* Palsies, Apoplexes, Diseases of that kind arising from cold humours; it breaketh Wind and easeth the Cholick.

The Dose is one spoonful at one time.

The Vertues of Spirit of Mint.

It is good for the Stomack, and strengthens the retentive Faculty, good against vomiting, and all Passions of the Heart, it comforteth the vital Spirits, and is good against the Consumption, it expelleth Wind, and helpeth Digestion, and is an infallible help for Melancholy.

The Dose is from one to two spoonfuls.

The Vertues of Aqua Theriacalis.

It is good against all Diseases of the Spleen whatsoever; It preventeth and helpeth Contagions, and sudden Oppressions and Qualms of the Heart.

The

The Dose is one spoonful to prevent, and three to the infected, who ought to sweat after taking it.

The Vertues of Spirit of Saffron.

It is good to comfort the vital Spirits, Passions, trembling, and pensiveness of the heart, and helpeth all Malignity oppressing it, and expelleth Wind, suppresseth fumes which arise from the Spleen, and go up to the head, and openeth the obstructions of it; it is excellent against all Melancholy, and very good for Women in Travel; for it comforteth and hasteneth delivery.

The Dose is morning and evening one spoonful for three days together.

Vertues of Spirit of Roses.

It is good to open the obstructions of the Lungs, and preventeth Consumptions, and other infirmities of that nature, it preserveth from putrifaction, and keepeth the breath from being corrupted.

The Dose is a spoonful at noon, at four in the afternoon, and as much at bed time.

The Vertue of the Spirit of Diasatyrion.

The Spirit made of *Diasatyrion magis gratum*, prescribed in the last *London* Dispensatory, comforteth and much restoreth decayed nature, strengtheneth the weak back, increaseth seed, and advanceth generation, being taken thrice a day a spoonful at a time, that is, in the morning fasting, at four in the afternoon, and last at bedward with this caution, that the weak parties abstain from venerial acts till after their first sleep.

The Dose is one spoonful at one time.

The Vertue of the Spirit of Strawberries.

It is excellent good to purifie and cleanse the blood; it preserveth from, and also cureth the yellow Jaundice, and deoppilateth the obstruction of the Spleen; It keepeth the body in a sweet temperateness, and refresheth the Spirits.

The Dose is a spoonful at a time, when need requireth any of those helps for the aforesaid Diseases.

Spirit of Confection of Alkermes Vertues.

It is an excellent Comforter of the Spirits vital, natural, and animal, in weak and delicate Persons, and against all trembling, pensiveness, and sudden qualms of the heart.

The dose is one spoonful at one time.

The virtue of Spirit of Comfry.

It hath all the virtues which Spirit of Clary hath, only it is of greater efficacy in inward hurts, bruises and ruptures.

The dose is one spoonful at one time.

Extract of Ambergriece.

Take a dram of Ambergriece, grind it very small on a Painters stone, then put it into a boult-head, then take of the best Spirit of Wine, either Canary, or Malligo Sack, half a pound, of Spirit of Clary, two ounces, mingle them well together, and pour of the Menstrua one pint to this proportion of Amber, set them to digest in a gentle Balneo about eight hours, shaking it together three or four times, then take it out, and being cold, pour it forth and put almost as much more of the mixed Spirits, digested as before in a gentle heat by Balneo, then put it forth to the first extracted; and and add half as much more Spirits the third time, and digest it again; and then have you extracted all the special part of the Amber, and leave nothing, but black dead earth of no value.

Then take a pint of the Spirit of what Herb you will use, and dissolve therein one pound of pure white Sugar-candy, or at the least twelve ounces, very finely powdered and searced through a fine Searcer, for the speedier Resolution thereof, it is best to dissolve it cold; this resolution must be twice filthered through a thin cap paper, to make it very perfect clear: then take three parts of this

dul-

dulcified Spirit, to one of your Extracts of Amber, drawn with Spirit of Wine, then shake them well together, and let them stand in a square glass very close stopped, until it shall be perfectly clear; one dram of this Extraction of Amber will serve to dulcify and make fit two quarts of Spirit of Mints, or Clary, or the like, and give it a most excellent taste and efficacious virtues.

Several Experiments made of the Countess of Kents, or of Gascons Powder, by a Professor of Physick.

1. A Child aged about five years, troubled much with flegm, and drawing on (as the Parents conceived) to his end, with ten grains of this powder, exhibited in a specifical vehicle, to the proportion of one spoonful, about seven of the clock at night, with the like dose exhibited the next morning, was within three days space perfectly recovered, and went abroad.

2. A Child aged about fourteeen years, being suddenly surprized with dangerous Fits, and trembling of the heart, with twelve grains of this Powder exhibited in a spoonful of *Aqua Theriacalis*, was that very day recovered.

3. A Stationers Child aged about five years, being suddenly taken so ill, that the Parents feared the life of the Child, with ten grains of this powder exhibited in a spoonful of Cordial Spirit, being laid down, and well covered (we suspected it would prove to be the small Pox) became within two or three hours somewhat chearful: And with this medicine continued once a day, the Pox broke forth, and the Child mended

4. A Boy aged about sixteen; being taken with suddain qualms about his stomach and heart, with ten grains of this powder exhibited in a spoonful of Doctor *Mountfords* water upon his fit, and the like quantity exhibited again when he went to bed, was the next day recovered.

K   5. A

5. A Child about three years old being troubled with grievous torments, and gripings in the belly with wind, with nine grains of this Powder, exhibited with two drops of specifical Oyl against the Cholick, in a spoonful of stomach Water, was eased in few hours.

6. A Child about seven years old, being troubled with Convulsion Fits, with ten grains of this Powder, mixed with Spirit of Castor, and one drop of Oil of Amber, in a few spoonfuls of black Cherry water, anointing the two neck veins near the ears, with a few drops of Oil of amber and Cloves, was suddenly recovered of his Fit.

7. A Gentlewoman, near forty years old, being oppressed with crude and flatuous humours, so that her friends thought her departing, was with twelve grains of this Powder, and two drops of a Cordial Oyl, exhibited in a spoonful of Cordial Water, being had to bed, within three days recovered, and followed her domestick business.

8. A Youth about twenty years old, much oppressed with wind and crudities of stomach, with twelve grains of this powder exhibited in two drops of specifical Cholick Oil, as in the fifth experiment, with a Cordial Water, was speedily recovered.

9. A Young Maid about eighteen years old, troubled with fits of the Mother, and Convulsive Fits, with twelve grains of this powder given her in a few spoonfuls of piony-water, gathered and distilled in due season, with a drop of oil of Cinnamon, and two of Amber mingled together, being held upright before a warm fire, within four hours recovered out of her fit, and went up to her chamber (though her teeth were set in her head, and small appearance of life) but that only her feet were warm, was discovered in her.

10. A Gentlewoman aged about fifty, being very

very much troubled with flatuous and crude humours oppressing the stomach, with sixteen grains of *Gascon* powder, and with three drops of Oil of Oranges, duly prepared, exhibited in an ounce of *Aqua Theriacalis*, being well shaken and mingled together, being exhibited at two several times, that is, at night when she went to bed, disposing for rest, and betimes the next morning, found much ease and comfort, and gained some quiet rest that night, and shortly recovered.

11. A Young Woman aged about four and twenty, not without some suspition of the plague, having a tumour long while arising on her groin, with three several doses of *Gascon* Powder, exhibited at three evenings when she disposed for rest, by twelve grains for every dose in a spoonful of triacle Water, drinking every morning a spoonful of Spirit of Saffron for those 3 days together, was perfectly recovered, and followed her domestick business.

These and many other experiments have I with good success tryed, and with Gods blessing recovered diverse several Patients.

This Powder is good against small Pox, Measels, spotted or purple Fever, exhibited in specifical Waters, fit for their several diseases; It is good in swouning and passions of the heart, arising from malignant vapours, or old causes, as also in the plague or pestilent Fevers, always observing to keep the persons upright, warm, and well covered after their taking it.

The dose of this powder in Children, is from eight to twelve grains, in persons more aged, from twelve to fourteen grains, but exhibite the dose twice or thrice if need require. In the plague you may use a greater quantity, with such medicines as are prescribed in the *Childs bearers Cabinet*, and it will not be amiss to mingle it with some *Aqua Theriacalis*.

The Composition of the Oil *called* Oleum Magistrale, *said to be invented by one named* Aparitius, *a Spaniard, being special good to cleanse and consoledate wounds, especially in the head.*

Take a quart of the best White-wine you can get, of pure old Oyl of Olives three pounds, then put thereto these flowers and herbs following, of the flowers and leaves of Hypericon half a pound, of *Carduus Benedictus,* of Valerian, of the least Sage of each a quarter of a pound, if it be possible, take the leaves and flowers of every one of these, then let them all steep twenty four hours in the aforesaid Wine and Oyl; the next day boil them in a pot well nealed, or in a copper vessel over a soft fire, until such time as the Wine be all consumed, stirring it always with a spattle; after you have thus done take it from the fire, and strain it, and put to the straining a pound and half of good *Venice* Turpentine, then boil it again upon a soft fire the space of a quarter of an hour, then put thereunto of Olibanum five ounces, of Myrrh three ounces, of *Sanguis Draconis* one ounce, and so let it boil till the Incense and Myrrh be melted, then take it off and let it stand until it be cold, then put it into a glass bottle, and set it eight or ten days in the Sun, and keep it for your use.

This Oil, the older it is, the better it is, it must be applied to the Patient wounded, as hot as may be endured, first washing the wound with White-wine, boiled with a handful of incense to comfort, and wiping it clean with a linnen cloth before you dress it, which must be, if it come to any brusings or bitings, twice a day, that is, about eight of the clock in the morning in winter and in summer about nine in the morning, and about four in the afternoon, but if they be green wounds you shall not need to change it again until the next day, neither need the Patient to observe any precise diet.

ADDITIONS.

A Rare Searcloth, with the Virtues.

Take of Oil-olive one pound and a half, red Lead one pound and a half, of white Lead one pound, Castle-sope four ounces, Oil of Bayes two ounces; put your Oil-Olive in a Pipkin, and put thereto your Oil of Bayes, and your Castle-sope; seeth these over a gentle fire of embers till it be well mingled, and melted together, then strew a little red Lead, and white, being mingled together in powder, still stirring it with a great spater of Wood, and so strew in more of your Lead by little and little till all be in, stirring it still by the bottom to keep it from burning for an hour and half together, then make the fire somewhat bigger, till the redness be turned into a gray colour, but you must not leave stirring it till the matter be turned into a perfect black colour as pitch; then drop a little upon a wooden Trencher, and if it cleave not to the Trencher, nor your Finger, it is enough; then take the long linnen cloaths, and dip them therein, and make your Sear-cloaths thereof: they will keep twenty years; let your powder of your Lead be searced very fine, and shred the Sope small.

The Virtues of this Sear-cloth, are:

Being laid to the Stomach it doth provoke Appetite, and taketh away any pain in the Stomach; being laid to the Belly, it is a present remedy for the Cholick, being laid to the Back, it is a present Remedy for the Flux, and running of the Reins, heat of the Kidneys, and weakness of the Back, it helpeth all Swellings and Bruises, taketh away Aches, it breaketh Fellons, and other Imposthumes, and healeth them; it draweth out any running humour,

mour, and helpeth him without breaking of the skin, and being applyed to the Fundament, helpeth any disease there; it helpeth all old Sores, and will be made in six hours.

For a Surfeit.

Take 3 pints of Muskadine, 1 handful of Rue, one handful of Red Sage; boil this together three or four walms: Take a quarter of an ounce of Nutmegs, half an ounce of Ginger, two or three corns of long Pepper; beat them all together, and boil them until the three pints comes to a quart: strain it, and put in it a quarter of an ounce of Methridate, half an ounce of London-triacle, a quarter of a pint of strong Angellica-water, all these being well mixed together, put them up into a Glass.

It is good for one that hath Surfeited to take three or four spoonfuls, keeping themselves very Warm in Bed; the same quantity taking is good against the Small-pox, or Measles.

It is good against the Wind, or pain in the Stomach, taking one spoonful in the Morning, or any Infection.

An Excellent Receipt against a Cough or a Consumption.

Take a quarter of a pound of the best Hony, a quarter of a pint of Conduit-water, boil them as long as any white scum ariseth, and take it off, then take a quarter of a pound of the best blew Currans, put them on the Fire in a pint of fair Water: Boil them until they be tender, then pour the Water from them, and bruise them through a hair Sieve, and put that Juice, and Hony together: Add to it one ounce of the powder of Liquorice, one ounce of the powder of Annise-seeds; mix all these together, and put them in a gally-pot, and when it is cold tye it up; the party troubled may take of it upon the point of a Knife Morning, or Evening, as often as the Cough taketh them.

Lucantellions Balsom, admirable for Wounds, and many other things.

Take of Venice Turpentine a pound, Oil-Olive three pints, yellow Wax half a pound, of natural Balsom one ounce, Oil of St Johns-wort one ounce, of red Saunders powdered an ounce, six spoonfuls of Sack: Cut the Wax and melt it on the Fire, and then left it catch the Fire, take it off, put in the Turpentine to it, having first washed the Venice-Turpentine thrice with Damask Rose-water, and having mingled your Sallade-Oil with the Sack, put also the Oil to them, and put them all on the Fire, and stir it till it begin to boil, for if it boil much it will run over speedily, then suffer it to cool for a night, or more, until the water and Wine be sunk all to the bottom, then make some holes in the stuff that the water may run out of it, which being done, put it over the Fire again, putting to it the Balsom, and the Oil of Saint Johns-wort; and when it is melted, then put the Sanders to it: Stir it well that it may Incorporate, and when it first begins to boil, take it off the Fire, and stir it the space of two hours, till it be grown thick, then put it up, and keep it for your use as most precious, for thirty or forty Years, or more.

The Virtues.

1. It is good to heal any wound inward or outward, being squirted warm into the inward Wound, being applyed to an outward Wound with fine lint, or linnen, anointing all those parts thereabouts, it not only taketh away the pain, but also keepeth it from any Inflammation, and also draweth forth all broken Bones, or any other thing that might putrifie or fester it, so that the Brains or Inwards, as the Liver, Guts, or part, be not touched, it will heal it in four or five days dressing, so that nothing be applied thereunto.

2. It also healeth any Burning or Scalding, and heal-

healeth alſo any Bruiſe or Cut, being firſt anointed with the ſaid Oil, and a piece of linnen cloth, or lint dipped in the ſame, being warmed and laid unto the Place it will heal it without any Scar remaining.

3. It helpeth the Head-ach by anointing the Temples and Noſtrils therewith.

4. It is good againſt the Wind Cholick, or ſtitch in the Side, applyed thereunto warm with hot clothes, morning and evening together, a quarter of an ounce.

5. It helpeth the biting of a mad Dog, or any other Beaſt.

6. It is good againſt the Plague, anointing only the Noſtrils, and the Lips therewith in the morning before you go forth.

7. It alſo healeth a Fiſtula, or Ulcer, be it never ſo deep in any part of the body, being applyed as aforeſaid is directed for a Cut.

8. It is alſo good againſt Worms, or Canker, being uſed as in a Cut, but it will require longer time to help them.

9 It is good for one infected with the Plague, Meaſles, ſo as it be preſently taken in warm Broth, the quantity of a quarter of an ounce four mornings together, and ſweat upon it.

10. It likewiſe helpeth Digeſtion, anointing the Navel and Stomack therewith when the Party goeth to Bed, it will ſtanch any Blood of a green Wound, put in a Plaiſter of lint on it, and tye it very hard.

11. The quantity of a Nutmeg in Sack bloodwarm, and ſweat thereon it, bringeth forth all manner of clotted Blood, and taketh away all Aches.

12. It alſo healeth the roſe Gout and Scurvy.

13 It helpeth all pains in Womens breaſts, all Chops or Wolf that cometh with a Bruiſe.

14 It helpeth the Small-pox, being anointed therewith without any Scar.

15. It

15. It helpeth all Sprains and Swellings, and indeed I cannot tell what comes amiss unto it.

A most certain and proved Medicine against all manner of Pestilence, and Plague, be it never so vehement.

Take an Onion, and cut it overthwart, then make a little hole in either piece, the which you shall fill with fine Triacle, and set the pieces together as they were before: after this wrap them in a fine wet linnen cloth, putting it to roast, and covered in the embers, or ashes, and when it is roasted enough, press out all the juyce of it, and give the Patient a spoonful, and immediately he shall feel himself better, and shall without fail be healed.

How to make the Ointment of Tobacco, Jobertus.

Take of green Tobacco-leaves two pound, of fresh Hogs-grease diligently wash'd one pound, bruise the herbs, and infuse it a whole night in red Wine, and then let it boil with the Hogs-grease on a gentle fire, until the Wine be all consumed: then strain it, and add to the Ointment the juyce of Tobacco one pound, good and clear Rosin four ounces, then boil it again till the juyce be consumed, adding towards the end, of round Birthwort-roots in powder two ounces, new Wax four ounces, or so much as is sufficient to make it into an Ointment.

The Virtues of it are these.

It cures all Tumors, Aposthumes, Wounds, Ulcers, Gun-shot, Botches, Itch, stinging with Nettles, Bees, Wasps, Hornets, or venemous Beasts, wounds made with poisoned Arrows, all Burnings and Scaldings, although it be with Oyl, or Lightning, and that without any Scar, it doth help all nasty, rotten, stinking, putrified Ulcers, although they be in the Legs where the humours be ready to resort most in Fistula's, although the bone be afflicted it will scale it without any Instrument, and bring up the flesh from the bottom; your Face being anoin-

anointed with it, it taketh away suddenly all Redness, Pimples, Sun-burnt; a Wound dressed with this Ointment, it will never putrify, it will cure a Wound when no Tent can searce it; it cures the Head-ach, the Temples being anointed therewith; the stomach being anointed with it, no infirmity will harbour there, no not Imposthumes, nor Consumption of the Lungs, the belly being anointed therewith; it helpeth the Chollick, and Illiack Passions, the Worms, (and what not) too tedious here to relate: it helpeth the Emeroids, or Piles, it is the best Ointment in the World for all sorts of Gouts whatsoever, and there can nothing come nigh unto it.

A very good Conserve for the help of a Consumption and Cough.

Take half a pound of blew Raisins, of the blackest sort is the best, and stone them, and skin them, and two ounces of white Sugar-candy, and two ounces of Oyl of sweet Almonds, and bruise them well, and when they be well incorporated together, use it to eat morning, noon, and night.

A very special Drink against a Consumption.

Take Colts-foot, Hysop, Scabious, and Maiden hair, of each a handful, and a quarter of a pound of Figs, and cut them in two pieces, and a quarter of a pound of Raisins, and stone them, and take ten Dates and stone them, and so boil them in four quarts of fair water, and after it hath boiled a little, put into it half an ounce of Liquorice scraped, and bruised, and so let it boil till one quart be boiled away, then take it off, and when it is cold strain it into a Pot, and drink half a pint each morning, at four of the Clock, and so much after Dinner at four of the Clock.

For Worms in Children.

Wormseed boiled in Beer or Ale, and then sweeten it with clarified Honey, and let them drink it.

How to drive away the Yellows of the Face that is caused by the overflowing of the Gall. Proved.

Take a great white Onion, and make a hole in the top of it, and then put into it the quantity of a Nutmeg of good Triacle, and then stop the hole again with the said piece that is cut out of it, but mingle the Triacle with Saffron powdered; this being done, roast the Onion in hot Embers, being wrapped up in wet Paper, and when it is well roasted wring out the Juyce thereof hard, and give the party this to drink in the Morning, and Sweat an hour after it, and so continue for three Mornings together, and then let the Party take a gentle Purge, & Fiat.

An Excellent Medicine for the Dropsie, made for Queen Elizabeth, by Doctor Adrian, *and Doctor* Lacy. *Proved.*

Take Polipodium, Spikenard, Squat, Ginger, Marjoram, Galingal, Setwel, *ana.* a penny weight, Sena leaves and cods, so much as all the rest grosly beaten; put them into a bag, and hang it in an earthen pot of two Gallons of Ale, and every four days cover the pot with new Barm, and drink no other drink for six Days, and this shall purge all ill Humors out of the Body, neither will it let the Blood putrify, nor flegm to have domination, nor Choller to burn, nor Melancholy to have exaltation, it doth encrease Blood, and helpeth all Evil, it helpeth and purgeth Rheum, it defendeth the Stomach, it preserveth the Body, and ingendereth good Colour, comforts the Sight, and nourisheth the Mind.

For the Dropsie that Swelleth.

Eat Water-cresses, and Raisins, use it often, and it will send down the Disease into the Legs and Feet, and when it is there, take the green bark of Elder in the Winter, and the crops in Summer, and boil them well in fair Water and Oat-meal to a Poultess, and apply it to the Grief, and this will Heal it.

The Celestial Water in the World for the Eyes.

Aqua *Celidonia,*
Aqua *Euphrasia,* } of each a quarter of a Pint.
Aqua *Finicula,*
Lapis *Tutia,* } of each a dram.
Lapis *Caluminaris,*

An Excellent Water for one that is near, or in a Consumption.

Take Milk three pints, red Wine one pint, twenty four Yolks of new-laid Eggs, beat them very well together, then add so much white Bread as will drink up the Wine, and put to it some Cowslip Flowers, and distil them, and take a spoonful first and last in Broth made of a Chicken, or Mutton, and in one Month it will Cure any Consumption.

For to stay Vomiting presently.

Take a little Mastick, and put it upon a hot Coal, and set a Funnel over it, and receive the fume into your Mouth, and let it go into your Stomach, & *Fiat.*

Doctor Teucables *green Balsom.*

Take in the Month of *May* Rosemary-tops, Wormwood, Balm, and Rue, *ana.* two ounces, red Sage, and Bay-buds, *ana.* four ounces, Sheepsfuet twelve ounces; beat all this very well together in a Stone Mortar, till it be all as a Salve, then put it into a clean Pipkin well stopt, and set it for eight days in a cold place, then put it all in a clean brass Chafer, and add to it a pound of Sweet Sallade-oil, and as many of the said Herbs as aforesaid well bruised, and let them boil over a soft fire very softly the space of an hour, and stir them all the time with a wooden Spatula, then take them from the fire, and presently put into it an ounce of Spike-oil, and stir them together, then with the

Spoon

Spoon take off the oily substance from the Herbs, and then strain it into a Gally-pot, and keep it very close stopt, and set it in a cool place, it will keep good two or three Years.

The Virtues are these.

The Virtue of the said Balm is in all Perfection good to cure all that is here under written, and the said Oyl is good to any Wounds either inward or outward; proved; being inward squirted into the said Wounds warm, and outward, being applyed with fine lint, or linnen, and anointing all the parts thereabouts.

1. It doth not only take away the pain, but it doth also keep it from Inflammation, and draweth forth also all broken Bones, or any thing else that might putrifie, or fester, if the Brains, Heart, Guts, Liver be not touched, it will heal in four or five times dressing, if no other thing be applyed thereunto.

It healeth any Burning or Scalding by fire, or water, or by any other means; it healeth any.

A Most excellent Powder much used by a person of Quality, lately Deceased; with the Virtues.

Take Pearl Magistrale prepared, Corral red and white prepared, prepared Amber, prepared Hartshorn, of each half an ounce, *Contra Yarva* one ounce; mingle them well together, then take three ounces of the black claws of Crabs before they be sodden, they must be taken in *June*, or *July*, the Sun being in *Cancer*, mingle all well together, then put to it four ounces of white Sugar-candy powdered, and mingle with the Sugar-candy, Ambergriece, Musk, Citron-seed skinned, *ana.* ten grains; beat the Seeds, Sugar-candy, and Amber-griece by themselves, very fine in a stone Mortar, all the rest must be passed through a fine Searce, then make a strong Jelly of Harts-horn, being boiled with White-wine, and infuse therein Saffron powdered

L two

two drams, and with this Jelly perfume the Powder, being all mixt into a paste, so make it up into little Balls, and set them into a warm Oven to dry, and then put them up to your use, the closer they be kept the better.

The Virtues of this Powder is most Excellent.

1. For to bring out the Small-pox, or if they be come out, take ten grains in Dragon-water each three hours, for nine hours.

2. For the Plague take ten grains in Dragon-water every three hours for nine hours, and sweat, and keep your self warm.

3. For a Heptick, take for nineteen days together, six grains every morning in Borrage-water.

4. For a Consumption, in Egrimony-water, take six grains for fourteen days together.

5. For the Cough of the Lungs, six grains, in half Bettony, and half Hysop-water, for fourteen days.

6. For any Ague or Fever, for three days, every third day take seven grains every three hours for nine hours in Carduus-water.

7. For Poison twelve grains boiled in a little Milk.

8. For a Woman that is sick after Labour, take seven grains every three hours for nine hours in Egrimony-water.

9. There is no Unicorns-horn comparable to it in contagious times, it is good to take five grains every morning in a little Sack.

10 For the Passion of the Heart, and Convulsion fits seven grains in Borrage-water, and it is a great Preserver of Health, working only as a Cordial, and you may safely take ten, twelve, fourteen, or sixteen, or eighteen, or twenty grains at once for a full Dose.

11. And if it be a great Feaver, small Pox, Plague, Poison, or for a Woman in Labour, put into

into every Dose three grains of Bezoar Oriental.

How to strengthen the Back, and to make one Lusty.

Take half a pint of Malmsey, and a handful of the pith of an Ox-back, but take the pith out from the skin, then take four or five stalks of Artechoaks, and take the pith out of them, but first cut the stalks into pieces so long as your finger, and then parboil them well, and take the pith from them, and then put it to the other things, and boil it gently to a Jelly, and when you have done so let it be cold, and then eat it upon the point of a knife morning and evening, and at any time of the day, so much as you shall think fitting, and if you would have it pleasant, make it sweet with white Sugar-candy, but not with Sugar.

For one that cannot make his Water.

Take Thyme and steep it in Wine-vinegar, one night or more, then take of this three spoonfuls, bloud-warm, after that you have eaten, at morning, noon, and night.

How to help a stinking Breath that cometh from the Stomach.

Take two handfuls of Cummin-seeds, and beat them to powder, and seeth it in a pottle of Whitewine, until half hath boiled away, and then give the party a good draught thereof first and last, morning and evening, as hot as he can suffer it, and in fifteen or sixteen days it will help.

For the Sciatica, or the Gout, my Lord of Sussex Medicine, called Flesh Unguentors.

Take of Rosin half a pound, of Perosin half a pound, of Virgins-wax four ounces, of Olibanum four ounces, of Mastick half an ounce, of Sheepstallow, or of Harts-tallow two ounces, of Camphire three drams, and of Turpentine three ounces.

The way to make it.

First beat all your Gums aforesaid every one by themselves, then take your Tallow and your Wax, and set them together on the fire, that done, put in your Rosin, then your Perosin, then your Olibanum, and last of all your Mastick; and when all is relented together over a soft fire of Coals, then strain it through a thin Canvas Cloth into a Pottle of White-wine, and then let them all boil together again until half the Wine be wasted and sod away; then take it from the fire, and let it cool, then afterward when it is almost cold anoint your hands with the Oyl of sweet Almonds, and work it up in Rouls like Wax-rouls, and in the time of the working thereof, cast in your Camphire beaten in fine Powder by it self alone; this observed that before you put in your Camphire into the Mortar for to be beaten into Powder, you must always beat in the same Mortar two or three Almonds, for else your Camphire will not be made into Powder.

The ordering of the same Medicine.

First you must spread it upon a fine linnen-cloth, plaister-wise, and so lay it upon every joynt where the pain is, but before the laying of your Plaister you must anoint all your Joynts with the Oyl of Roses, and the stuff of your Plaister must be half an inch thick, and according unto the Property of the same you must let it stick and cling where you lay it for the space of nine or ten days together, notwithstanding it doth put you to some pain or itch in the mean time, yet you must in any-wise let it lie on still, for it will both draw out the sinews by little small Pimples, and also heal it again, and this one Plaister must serve during all the time of your Disease without any manner of renewing.

Prob. of Witness by my Lo.d of *Suffolk*.

A